Love, Zac

Love, Zac

Small-Town Football and the Life and Death of an American Boy

REID FORGRAVE

ALGONQUIN BOOKS
OF CHAPEL HILL   2020

Published by
Algonquin Books of Chapel Hill
Post Office Box 2225
Chapel Hill, North Carolina 27515-2225

a division of
Workman Publishing
225 Varick Street
New York, New York 10014

Library of Congress Cataloging-in-Publication Data

Names: Forgrave, Reid, [date]– author.
Title: Love, Zac / small-town football and the life and death of
an American boy / Reid Forgrave.
Description: Chapel Hill, North Carolina :
Algonquin Books of Chapel Hill, [2020] |
Summary: "The story of a young man from small-town Iowa who
decided to take his own life rather than continue his losing battle against the
traumatic brain injuries (CTE) he had sustained as a no-holds-barred high
school football player, and at the same time a larger story about the hot-button
issues that football raises about masculinity and violence, and about what
values we want to instill in our kids"— Provided by publisher.
Identifiers: LCCN 2020016842 | ISBN 9781616209087 (hardcover) |
ISBN 9781643751092 (e-book)
Subjects: LCSH: Easter, Zac, 1991–2015. | Football players—Iowa—Biography. |
High school athletes—Iowa—Biography. | Football injuries—Patients—
Iowa—Biography. | Brain—Concussion—Patients—Iowa—Biography.
Classification: LCC RC1220.F6 F68 2020 | DDC 617.1/027092 [B]—dc23
LC record available at https://lccn.loc.gov/2020016842

10 9 8 7 6 5 4 3 2 1
First Edition

To Megan, the one I want to impress

Contents

Love, Zac

Prologue

ZAC EASTER STOOD on the long wooden dock leading out onto Lake Ahquabi, gripping the .40-caliber pistol he'd given his dad for Father's Day not even five months before.

The sun had dipped over the horizon on the other side of the Y-shaped lake. Leaves lay in heaps on the fringe of the woods. The gusty November winds died down as the sun sank on the horizon, but there was still a chill in the air. Winter was coming. Zac took out his phone and snapped a picture. He posted it to Snapchat, ignoring the frantic phone calls that were pouring into his phone. God bless America, he captioned the photo.

Where is Zac? All around Zac's hometown, friends and family were terrified. They'd seen his Facebook post a few minutes before: "If your reading this than God bless the times we've had together. Please forgive me. I'm taking the selfish road out. Only God understands what I've been through . . . I will always watch over you!"* They needed to stop him. But how? They didn't even know where he was. From the house where Zac grew up, a few miles away and amidst fields of corn, his parents called. Zac did not pick up. From the small town just down the street where Zac

---

* Zac's often-haphazard spelling is retained when quoting from his diary and other writings.

had played high school football, and from Des Moines, the big capital city not quite twenty miles to the north, his friends called. Zac did not pick up. At 5:36 p.m., a college roommate texted him: "Hey what're you up to bud?" No reply. From the law school at Case Western Reserve University, almost seven hundred miles away in Cleveland, Ohio, Ali Epperson—Zac's girlfriend, and the only person to whom he had fully confided his struggles with his rapidly deteriorating brain—called. Zac did not pick up.

She called again.

He did not pick up.

She called again.

Finally, Zac picked up. There was terror in his voice.

"I can't do this," he told her. "It's never going to get better."

Ali, a vivacious law student who in many ways was Zac's opposite—a bleeding-heart liberal who balanced out Zac's dyed-in-the-wool conservatism—was freaking out. How many hours had she spent on the phone with him, talking about the disease that seemed to be eating his brain from the inside? How many times had the two talked about the sport he loved, the sport that had consumed much of his childhood but now seemed to be consuming the rest of his life as well? How many times had she told him that a real man was not stoic and unfeeling—that a real man must face his demons instead of suffering silently in deference to some antiquated ideal of masculinity? How many times had she told him not to apologize to her, that she loved him despite the crazy stuff that was going on, and that they would work through it all together?

Earlier on this day—Friday the 13th, of all days, in November 2015—he had apologized again. "I'm sorry you fell in love with a guy with a ducked up brain," Zac had texted her, his phone's autocorrect softening the swear word. He'd awoken early, started drinking, and called Ali in a panic late in the morning, shit-faced and swerving his car around the suburbs. She'd coaxed him to drive into a gas station, then into a Jimmy John's to grab a sandwich and sober up. She'd calmed him like she always did. He'd apologized like he always did. She'd texted him back: "You can't choose who you fall in love with. You just fall in love." Then, he'd texted an ominous reply: "If anything happens to [me] just by a chance of luck. Tell my family everything."

Now, things were happening. A friend noticed the setting of Zac's Snapchat photo: the beach on Lake Ahquabi, where Zac and Ali had escaped to in the summer to get away from high school friends and stare at the clouds. The lake was just down the road from his family's house. The lake's name is derived from an ancient Algonquian language. It means "resting place."

Ali kept Zac on the phone. "Listen to the sound of my voice," she soothed him. "Listen to the sound of my voice."

"I'm losing my mind," he cried. "This is it for me!" One Warren County Sheriff's Office cruiser came speeding down the winding hill toward the lake, followed by another. "Ali, did you send these cops here?" The cops got closer to him. He started apologizing to Ali, and he told her he wanted his brain donated for research. Then, Zac's phone cut out.

Out on the dock, Zac pointed the pistol at the darkened sky and fired a warning shot.

That is when a pickup truck sped down the hill and slammed to a stop next to the lake. Zac's father, a burly former high-school football coach named Myles Easter, jumped out. The parking lot quickly filled with squad cars. One deputy, a former all-conference linebacker who played for Myles on the same high school team Zac had played for, trained his assault rifle on Zac. Lasers from other police rifles danced on Zac's body. The evening was dark, and it was getting cold. Myles saw the cherry-red 2008 Mazda3 Zac called Old Red. He peered into the window of his son's car. He saw an empty six-pack of Coors Light, an empty bottle of Captain Morgan rum, and a pill bottle.

Floodlights illuminated Zac. A black curtain fell on the water behind him. Zac stood up from a picnic table and walked down the pier toward a wooden fishing hut at water's edge. A few more steps, and he'd be inside, alone on the water, out of sight.

"Put your gun down!" the deputies shouted.

"Nope!" Zac yelled with an anguished laugh. "Not gonna do that!"

In a flash, Zac's father realized what was happening: *Zac wants the police to shoot him.* "Fuck it," Myles said to himself. "I can't let this happen."

Zac's father sprinted past the sheriff's deputies and onto the pier. "Zac!" he shouted. *If he shoots me, he shoots me*, the father thought.

"Dad, stop!"

As Myles Easter ran toward his son, Zac's face came into focus. His blue eyes looked foggy and confused. The expression on his still-boyish face matched the tenor of his voice: sad, sick, exhausted, scared. Worn down by life. Beaten, once and for all.

"Zac, I'm coming," Myles said. "Put your gun down."

"Dad!" Zac shouted. "Dad, stop!"

Then, gripping his father's pistol, Zac disappeared into the fishing hut. The door slammed shut behind him.

And Zac Easter was alone.

ONE

The Seed

IOWA'S CAPITOL BUILDING sits on a grassy hill just east of downtown Des Moines. It marks the highest point on the east side of this Midwestern city. Atop the rectangular limestone structure, four smaller copper domes encircle one large dome in the center, which ascends 275 feet above the ground. The large dome is gilded with 150 troy ounces of 23-karat gold leaf. Six intimidating Corinthian columns rise up on each side of the building to ornately designed cornices at the roofline. The architectural message from this enormous edifice, for which the cornerstone was laid in 1871, seems to be this: Respect authority. Nearby is a newly hopping entertainment district that a little more than a decade before had a reputation somewhere between sketchy and abandoned.

Across two parking lots and past an office building is the busy US Highway 69. Get on it and go south: over the Des Moines River, past the car dealerships and the RV dealerships and the mobile home parks and the cheap motels. Pass the car washes and the immigrant-owned small businesses and the storage lockers. Pass the Home Depot and the Walmart Supercenter and the miles of suburban chain restaurants. Soon, the highway hangs left then swings back to the right, and the hills become rolling, the cornfields and forests vast, the chain stores and restaurants gone, the houses much fewer and farther between. I made this drive dozens of times while I lived in Iowa. It was always a calming feeling, the city melting away as rural America opened up before me.

The skies are boundless. Christ Died For Our Sins, 1 Corinthians, reads a road sign. There are silos and grain bins, machine sheds and water towers. There's an ad for a Harley Davidson dealership and a sign for a shooting range. Then, for a dozen miles, there's not much but farm fields, filled with corn and soybeans in the state's rich, silty soil that people here call black gold. This soil is what makes Iowa the place people mean when they talk about the nation's breadbasket, a place disparaged or just plain forgotten about by the coasts but vital to the nation's survival, and to its fractured and diverse national culture. A local clothing store sells a T-shirt with a map of the United States and an arrow pointing to the middle of the country. IOWA, the shirt reads. WAVE THE NEXT TIME YOU FLY OVER!

The highway rises and falls, and soon buildings appear again. A Buick GMC car dealership. Calvary Baptist Church. Newly built suburban developments interrupting those endless miles of farm fields. A meat locker, a bait shop. Three huge cement towers that can store more than two million bushels of grain at Heartland Co-op's facility. The Harley Davidson dealership, right next door to the John Deere dealership. And the National Balloon Museum, a reminder of what Indianola is best known for: a huge annual nine-day hot-air balloon festival each summer, during which nearly a hundred colorful hot-air balloons paint the Iowa skies.

On the edge of this town of sixteen thousand residents, a half hour's drive from the Iowa capital, a small sign—Indianola, Est. 1849—welcomes you to the place where Zac Easter was raised.

Every four years, Iowa becomes a national caricature. Presidential candidates trot through the state to prove themselves worthy during the first-in-the-nation presidential caucuses. Iowans like to joke that for one month every four years, the rest of the nation cares about Iowa's problems. Then, Iowans cast their votes, and the nation moves on. On national television news, Iowa is presented as a state of seed-corn hats and hay bales, Carhartt bib overalls and pork-chops-on-a-stick. But the character of this state makes it less a rural anomaly than a bellwether of the Midwest. As a transplant from the East Coast, I found Iowa an understated place, where people are less prone to shouting and more prone to understanding, and where natural beauty can be found not in snowcapped mountains or crashing ocean waves but in the quiet serenity of a summer breeze rustling over a soybean field. And it is a place where the values of the sport of football—of hard work and teamwork, of a community that rallies around a cause, of a faith that each of us is but a small, vital piece in a much grander plan—align perfectly with the values of everyday life.

Now, leave the small town of Indianola and head a few miles into the country. Today is the day of the Iowa Hawkeyes' spring scrimmage, and the university's head football coach is talking on the radio. Like a mellower version of football-mad Alabama, the broadcast of the exhibition game reaches throughout the state of Iowa. As Iowa's coach speaks about the returning players who make up his team's beefy offensive line, drive past the graveyard, past the huge hay bales splotched on coffee-colored fields, past the farm pond where a rowboat is tied to a dock. Cows lounge near a rusting silo. The pavement stops, and the road turns to gravel. A sign reads: HAY FOR SALE. The hills climb and dive

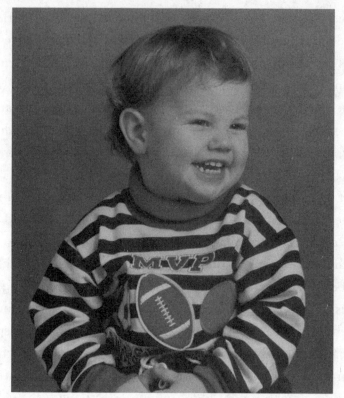

Zac as a toddler

next to rows of newly planted corn, an antique windmill, and whitewashed fences that keep in the horses. A teenage boy zips by on his four-wheeler, heading from his family's goat farm toward their house. A cloud of dust encircles you as you turn onto 92nd Lane. A few houses in, on five wooded acres of timber, sits the Easter household, the place where Zac Easter, all-American boy, grew into a man.

They called him Hoad. On Saturday mornings, the three young Easter boys—Myles II was the eldest, then Zac, then Levi—would crowd around the television to watch *Garfield and Friends*. In the cartoon, Odie was the mutt who was Garfield's best friend. With floppy ears and a tongue that constantly hung out, he was honest, kind, and impossibly energetic. Friends with everyone, he was mischievous yet lovable. A bit goofy, sure, but a truly decent being through and through. And all that stuff about Odie? That was Zac, too. "Zac never stopped running. Everything he did was at full charge," said his mother, Brenda Easter. Over time the name evolved, the way nicknames do—Odie morphing into Hodie, Hodie shrinking to Hoad.

Zac was a sweet, curious kid, always sporting a smile but seemingly programmed to destroy. At eighteen months, he climbed up the curtains, grabbed his grandmother's prized china egg, dropped it, and broke it. As a kid, he went through four of those supposedly unbreakable steel Tonka dump trucks. He broke the first three and then, at age seven, disassembled the fourth, his boundless curiosity spurring him to figure out how the toy worked. At age eight, when an ambulance rushed by his house, siren blaring, Zac pretended to crash his bicycle to see if the ambulance would stop. (It didn't.) The dimpled, boyish face that followed Zac until adulthood seemed to easily get him out of trouble: *Who, me?* The mischief was mostly harmless but always there. One winter, the family couldn't figure out why the light bulbs on the Christmas tree kept bursting. Faulty wiring? Time to invest in new Christmas lights? Nope. Turned out the cause was Zac, taking swings at the bulbs with a baseball bat.

As he got older, the blast radius got bigger. In the woods surrounding his home, he was Tom Sawyer reborn: undiluted, unleashed, Midwestern middle-class American *boy*. The Easter family's acreage was just east of a piece of land made somewhat famous for its antique covered bridges—the part of the world where *The Bridges of Madison County* was filmed. Zac and his friends would head into the woods to play soldier, shooting one another with the plastic pellets of Airsoft toy guns, pretending to be the military heroes of movies they loved like *Platoon* or *The Deer Hunter*. He and his brothers would go on hikes to the creek, bringing along an artillery of Black Cat fireworks to blow up minnows and bullfrogs. (An unspoken agreement among Zac's high school friends was that anytime anybody made a trip through neighboring Missouri, where fireworks could be purchased legally, they'd return with $100 or $200 worth of fresh ordnance.) As a teenager, he graduated to the family's Honda Recon ATV, his first taste of real adrenaline, and real recklessness, too. He'd fly through the woods, bank on two wheels, and carve the tightest, fastest semicircles he could. He'd build jumps and hurtle over them. Zac knew these trails by heart. He could almost ride them with his eyes closed. "GODDAMMIT!" his dad would yell from the porch as he watched Zac's close-cropped chestnut hair zip by. And Zac, as always, just kept going. "He really was reckless on that, just wild," his father later recalled. "He was confident he wouldn't wreck, always in control. Honestly, that's what you want on a football team, too."

You weren't a real member of the Easter family if you didn't love guns. The three boys joined their dad on hunts starting when they were five or six. At age nine, each received his first firearm; by that point the boy was trained in gun safety and itching to shoot. The oldest son, Myles II, bagged a six-point buck his very first hunt with his dad. Levi, the youngest, would eventually become the best shot of the three. There was a rhythm to the family's hunting trips: sitting in the tree stand, soaking in the silence, then moving around to rustle deer out from the woods. They'd spread out to be alone, keeping in contact with cell phones, and then they'd get back together. Always they kept an eye out for rattlesnakes.

At the edge of the family's backyard is where the tree line begins. Every night, the boys' father would grab a shotgun and a pistol, rustle up the family's two rat terriers, Tito and Max, and go for a walk in the woods. Not a *walk*, really. More of a prowl. Myles Easter was looking for targets. Every January he tacks a new blank sheet of paper to the refrigerator. At the top of the sheet are the words *KILL LIST*. By the end of the year, the kill list is typically filled with more than a hundred animals: deer, squirrels, snakes, muskrats. He takes the list so seriously that he has placed several motion-activated trail cameras out there, so he'll know if a prized big buck, or something even more exotic, has crept into the Easters' territory. The boys would join their dad on his backyard hunts as well as hunts on the family land nearby. The best hunts would enter into family lore—or, with a perfectly placed shot and a bit of luck, onto a sacred spot on the wall in their living room with its vaulted ceiling. There, the family's top kills lived on for eternity—the animals staring out from the two-story whitewashed drywall, with the help of taxidermy.

One of the favorite Easter family hunting stories dates back to when Zac was a teenager. He and his father spotted a rabbit in the backyard. Zac raced inside and grabbed a .50-caliber muzzle-loader, a huge rifle fit more for the Wild West era than the twenty-first century. Zac being Zac, he ran back outside and jammed way too much gunpowder into the rifle. He fired: *BOOM!* Their ears rang. Pieces of rabbit flew up to the tree line, with a bunny carcass spinning in the air. The Easter men couldn't stop laughing for the rest of the night. Brenda Easter just sighed. This was her life as the only woman in a home of four testosterone-juiced men.

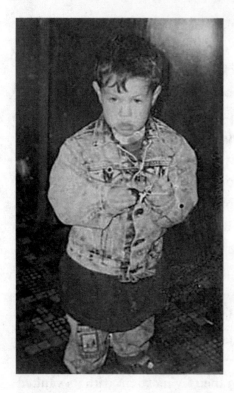

Zac as a young boy.

A forty-minute drive away is the Easter family timber, some eighty acres of wooded hills that aren't suitable for farming. What they are suitable for is world-class deer hunting. And from the first day of deer season until the last each year—from right after Thanksgiving until right after New Year's—Myles Easter and his three boys would spend every free moment roaming the family land. They would wake up well before sunrise, and Myles would cook up a breakfast of bacon and eggs. They'd jump into his Ford pickup and drive to the timber, sipping coffee the entire way. Sometimes they got a deer. Sometimes they didn't. Either way— from when he was a young boy until he was a college graduate— these were the happiest days of Zac Easter's life.

Two things mattered most among the Easter men. The first was hunting. The second was football. Zac's father had fallen in love with the sport as a youth and dedicated much of his life to it, as a high school and college coach as well as his sons' biggest supporter. And football was something that Zac Easter seemed perfectly attuned to. The sport captured the imagination of all three Easter boys almost from the womb. But Zac was fearless, the toughest dude around.

In Zac's developing young mind, he was more superhero than human. Zac Easter, you see, believed he was invincible. He was confident he could push his limits to the very edge yet always stay in control. His ethos was a controlled type of chaos. He was never the most gifted athlete on the field, and his body wasn't the best suited for the sport. He worked on his physique, spending hours upon hours in the gym. Compared to the more hulking players, however, he was still fairly small. But it wasn't his body that mattered as much as his mind. The way he thought—or the way he often *didn't* think, instead throwing all caution into the wind— meant that he could beat you through sheer force of will because he was willing to take a risk with his body that you weren't willing to take.

Zac Easter's brain, it seemed, had been put on this earth to play football.

THE MOMENT WHEN football fully captured the American imagination can be hard to pinpoint. We can definitively say that the seed of our national obsession was first planted in Brunswick, New Jersey, on November 6, 1869, four years after the end of the Civil War and the assassination of President Abraham Lincoln, when Rutgers and Princeton (then known as the College of New Jersey) played a sport that was a derivative of rugby. It was later billed as the first collegiate football game. (Rutgers won, 6–4.) But it wasn't like the game of football was invented one year and had spread like wildfire by the next. The history of football, that most violent and disciplined of sports, progressed in fits and starts, and for most of its first few decades, it was played in the shadow of the more bucolic American pastime of baseball.

What we can say with absolute certainty today is that a century and a half after the sport was conceived, football has become an essential part of the American landscape and distilled the American psyche (in all its contradictory complexity) more than any other sport. The NFL has reached $15 billion in annual revenue, a number that is greater than the gross domestic product of some seventy countries and the largest of any sports league in the world. If the NFL were a publicly traded entity—legally, it considers itself a trade association with the thirty-two team owners functioning as its shareholders—it would rank among the top two hundred companies in America in terms of revenue, in the same ballpark as Visa, General Mills, and the Marriott hotel chain.

And that's only the professional version of the sport. The twenty-five most valuable college football programs bring in $2.5 billion in revenue annually, and *Forbes* reported in 2019 that the most profitable collegiate team, the Texas A&M Aggies, brought in an average of $147 million in annual revenue over the past three years. When the new College Football Playoff held an auction for twelve years of television rights, ESPN's winning bid came to $7.3 billion. That's $7.3 *billion* for the right to televise just seven games a year for a dozen years. As Gilbert M. Gaul noted in his book *Billion-Dollar Ball: A Journey through the Big Money of College*

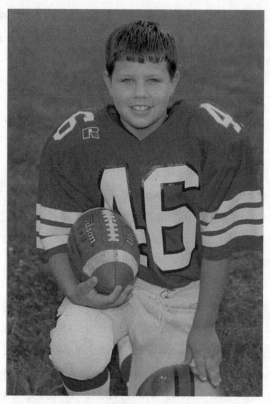

*Zac started youth football in third
grade, his father as coach.*

Football, the football program at the University of Texas has a
higher profit margin than ExxonMobil or Apple. More than a million Americans play high school football annually, a number that's
dwarfed by the estimated seventy-five million Americans who play
so-called fantasy football, which involves fans choosing individual
players for their "team" and using those players' statistics to compete against friends' teams to win money.

A few decades ago, it was reasonable to argue whether baseball
or football was the favorite American pastime. This argument can

no longer be honestly debated. Football has become less of a sport and more of an ingrained feature of American life. As a character in the Will Smith film *Concussion* put it so memorably: "The NFL owns a day of the week. The same day the Church used to own. Now, it's theirs." In modern-day America, football is as much religion as sport.

But when was football's tipping point? In those 150-some years between that day when a hundred or so people attended the Rutgers–College of New Jersey game of 1869 and the modern-day spectacle of 114.4 million Americans (more than a third of the US population) tuning in to see the New England Patriots defeat the Seattle Seahawks, 28–24, in Super Bowl XLIX on February 1, 2015, in the most-watched television broadcast in American history, at which point did football first solidify its iron grip on the American sporting imagination? Was it in 1880, when collegiate teams at the College of New Jersey and Yale decided to stage a contest of this new and exciting and most importantly *American* sport in New York City on Thanksgiving Day, turning this revered national holiday into a spectacle of sport? Was it when President Teddy Roosevelt threatened in 1905 to ban the game, which led to rule reforms and the formation of the National Collegiate Athletic Association, giving the sport an organizational structure? Was it when the forward pass was invented, which helped American football evolve beyond rugby to become a far more exciting, multifaceted game of military-like strategy? Was it the development of star professional players such as Jim Thorpe and Bronko Nagurski? Or was it during the 1972 playoffs when the Pittsburgh Steelers' Franco Harris caught an errant ball and ran it in for a touchdown in one of the most famous plays in NFL history, which came to be known as the Immaculate Reception?

While each of these were defining moments in the sport's march from a savage and unorganized game that was really little more than hazing for college freshmen to this national religion, none can quite stack up to the impact of the game that was played on December 28, 1958. It's fitting that this game happened at Yankee Stadium, "The House That Ruth Built." Football marched into the most iconic baseball venue in the world and proclaimed during this one stormy afternoon in the Bronx that it, not baseball, was the new king of American sports. It was the NFL championship game between the workmanlike New York Giants and the much more glamorous Baltimore Colts, and it was watched by forty-five million fans nationwide on NBC. It featured names that would become synonymous with the sport over the next half century: The Colts' quarterback was Johnny Unitas, nicknamed "the Golden Arm" and still considered one of the greatest quarterbacks to ever have played the game. The Giants' running back was Frank Gifford, whose Hall of Fame football heroics were later surpassed by the celebrity that came with a twenty-seven-year career as a broadcaster for ABC's *NFL Monday Night Football*—and who was posthumously diagnosed with the same degenerative brain disease that befell Zac Easter.

Manning the sidelines for the Giants were two assistant coaches who were little known at the time but would soon become icons of the game. One was defensive assistant coach Tom Landry, who'd go on to coach "America's Team," the Dallas Cowboys, for twenty-nine years and win two Super Bowls in the process. The other was offensive assistant coach Vince Lombardi, who would become one of the most admired coaches in American sports history as he led the Green Bay Packers to win the first two Super Bowls, in 1967 and 1968. Lombardi's aphorisms became synonymous with the machismo culture of both football and postwar America: "It's not whether you get knocked down—it's whether you get up." "The man who wins is the man who thinks he can." "If you can walk, you can run. No one is ever hurt. Hurt is in your mind." Nearly fifty years after Lombardi's untimely death in 1970, Zac Easter would make the seven-hour pilgrimage from his family's home in Iowa to the famous frozen tundra of Lambeau Field in Green Bay, Wisconsin. The Packers were his favorite team. And Lombardi was his favorite coach. Even though others in his family were fans of one of the Packers' rivals, the Minnesota Vikings, what Lombardi stood for—toughness, dedication, and stoicism as the traits that define manhood—was powerful enough that it warranted a framed Lombardi photo hanging in the Easters' basement.

The Colts-Giants championship game on that cold, blustery December afternoon in 1958 was a historic sporting battle. As Michael MacCambridge detailed in his book *America's Game: The Epic Story of How Pro Football Captured a Nation*, it was a back-and-forth fight from the opening kickoff, filled with exciting miscues and jaw-dropping plays. Unitas fumbled on the Colts' first drive, but on the very next play the Giants' quarterback Don Heinrich fumbled the ball right back to the Colts. Not to be outdone in the quarterbacking struggles, the future Hall of Famer Unitas promptly threw another interception. On the Colts' next drive, Unitas seemed to have the Colts heading in the right direction when he completed a sixty-yard pass to Lenny Moore, but then Giants linebacker Sam Huff, one of a record seventeen future Hall of Famers involved in this game, blocked the Colts' field goal attempt.

By the end of the first half, after Unitas threw a fifteen-yard touchdown pass to Raymond Berry, the Colts held a 14–3 lead. At the beginning of the third quarter, after the Colts turned the ball over at the one-yard line on the doorstep of a big touchdown, the Giants pulled off one of the most exciting plays in NFL history. Charlie Conerly, who had replaced Heinrich as the Giants' quarterback, took the snap deep in his own territory. He faked a hand-off, and it looked like a broken play as Gino Marchetti, the Colts' hulking defensive end from a coal-mining town in West Virginia, broke past blockers and ran straight at Conerly. Conerly threw an off-balance pass from his back foot as the Colts' lineman jumped in his face. Somehow, the pass made it to midfield, where Giants wide receiver Kyle Rote caught the ball, shed a tackle, and then streaked toward the end zone. At the twenty-five-yard line, Rote was hit from behind. He fumbled, but the fumble was improbably picked up by Giants running back Alex Webster, who ran it all the way to the one-yard line. The Giants scored on the next play, and momentum swung their way.

Nobody could turn their heads from the drama on the field. Marchetti broke his ankle during a play in the fourth quarter, but he wouldn't leave the field to get it treated. By this point, his Colts were losing, 17–14, with just under two minutes left in the game. Marchetti watched from a stretcher on the sidelines as Gifford nearly made a first down, a gain that would have sealed the game for the Giants. But referees controversially ruled Gifford was down before the first-down marker, and the Colts had a chance to tie things up. Unitas methodically marched his Colts down the field, and they tied up the game with a field goal from the thirteen-yard line with seven seconds left. At his family's home in New York, six-year-old Bob Costas stared at the television in wonder as the game went into overtime. It was the first sporting event the future sportscasting legend remembers watching on television.

It wasn't just because it was a one-game spectacle that Costas and millions more Americans would remember this NFL championship game for as long as they lived. It was because they were witnessing, in real time, this sport claim its dominion over modern American culture.

The modern age was synonymous with post–World War II corporate America. The undisputed victor of the war, the United States saw a prosperity boom after 1945, and participating in and viewing sports, whether live or on television, became a preferred way to spend that extra cash and free time. What's more, football seemed perfectly suited to a generation of soldiers who had returned from the battlefields of World War II: Veterans valued the discipline, violence, and game planning that has long made football the most militaristic of sports. In fact, football is in many ways a sporting allegory for the type of land-grabbing wars that marked the rise of human civilizations. Think of how football works: One team is trying to gain ground on another team. A group of blockers—*foot soldiers* who do their work in the *trenches*—clear the path for the team to move the ball forward. A quarterback is called a *field general*. The passing game is called the *air attack*, a long pass called a *bomb*, a short pass a *bullet*. Multiple defensive players rushing headlong at the quarterback is a *blitz*, stemming from the German military's *blitzkrieg* of World War II. When both teams line up before a snap, they're lining up in *formations*. As the military-industrial complex built up during the Cold War, the militaristic, us-versus-them nature of football played right into the American psyche. It is not just some coincidence that eleven days after the beginning of the first Gulf War in January 1991, Super Bowl XXV was infused with patriotism: from Whitney Houston's galvanizing rendition of the national anthem, to the tiny American flag each fan was given upon entering Tampa Stadium, to the taped halftime address by President George H. W. Bush, during which he referred to the Gulf War as his Super Bowl. If the writer George Orwell once referred to Olympic and international sports as "war minus the shooting," then football is that view's apotheosis.

But there was another aspect of football that was on display during that NFL championship game three days after Christmas in 1958: the power of television. Televisions were becoming ubiquitous in American households during the 1950s. In 1948, 172,000 American households had televisions, but by 1950, nearly four million American homes did. A decade later that number was a stunning forty-six million, more than a tenfold increase. And at a time when America was primed for a sport with a national following instead of the more regionalized sport of baseball, there was no better sport for television than the back-and-forth pitched horizontal battles of football. As James Michener noted in his book *Sports in America*, football and television have an "almost symbiotic" relationship. By the 1970s, the Super Bowl would become an unofficial holiday, and announcers like Frank Gifford and Howard Cosell would become celebrities.

While televisions fueled the growth of football, they affected baseball in the opposite fashion. In 1948, shortly after televisions were introduced to a mass American audience, baseball's live attendance was twenty-one million. Five years later, in 1953, that attendance had dipped dramatically, to 14.3 million, as more and more baseball-loving Americans chose to stay home and watch the games from the comfort of their sofas instead of heading to the ballpark. Meanwhile, television actually proved a boon to live football attendance: Average attendance nearly doubled from 1949 to 1959. Baseball is an individual's game, more suited to America's agrarian past. As America moved into a less individualistic, more regimented future, football—more militaristic, more group oriented, more corporate—took over.

But as the 1958 championship game went into the first sudden-death overtime ever in an NFL playoff game, tens of millions of Americans got to witness the precarious side of live television. A moment after the twenty-five-year-old Unitas completed a twelve-yard pass to Raymond Berry for a first down at the Giants' eight-yard line, a win firmly within the Colts' grasp, American television viewers were treated to an infuriating message on their television screens. At the height of the drama, their televisions turned to black. "Please Stand By" read a message on the screens, at the most inopportune of times. "PICTURE TRANSMISSION HAS BEEN TEMPORARILY INTERRUPTED." In Yankee Stadium, NBC officials panicked. They quickly identified the problem: Rowdy and excited Colts fans next to the field had accidentally disconnected a cable, which cut out the television signal. But the game was still going on.

Until, that is, a drunk sprinted onto the field. The whistle blew, and the game was halted. Three New York City cops wrestled the drunk to the ground. He was arrested, and play eventually resumed. Fortunately, enough time had passed during the interruption that NBC officials were able to reconnect the television cable and continue the broadcast. It wasn't until later that it was revealed the "drunk" was actually an NBC business manager who had purposefully run onto the field to delay the game, the very definition of taking one for the team.

The television broadcast flickered back on. The afternoon skies were darkening under the Yankee Stadium lights as Colts running back Alan Ameche was stuffed for a one-yard run. Then, Unitas completed a six-yard pass to tight end Jim Mutscheller, putting the Colts at the one-yard line for a critical third-down play. Unitas handed the ball off to Ameche again. Ameche was a swarthy, dark-haired twenty-five-year-old from Wisconsin who'd won the Heisman Trophy in college for the University of Wisconsin. He was nicknamed "the Iron Horse," and he lived up to the moniker on that play. He took the handoff, ran slightly to his right, and dove over a defender who awaited him at the goal line. The Colts had won what would become known as the greatest game ever played. Baltimore fans ran onto the field and tore down the goalposts. Ameche went into Manhattan to be a guest on that night's *The Ed Sullivan Show*, which a little more than five years later would present the Beatles and thereby launch another American cultural sea change: the all-encompassing takeover of rock 'n' roll. In Baltimore, a crowd of thirty thousand fans awaited the victorious team at Friendship Airport that night, bringing traffic on the highway to a near standstill.

Football was no longer "Savagery on Sunday," as a 1955 *Life* magazine cover had proclaimed. That story just a few years earlier had displayed some moral ambivalence about the rise of such a violent sport. After the 1958 championship game, *Life* tweaked its wording when it wrote about football, still calling the sport a "celebration of savagery" but recognizing that there was something about that violence that Americans adored: "an audience eager to embrace savagery as heroic." A *Time* magazine cover in 1959 about the explosion of football featured a photo of Sam Huff and the headline "A Man's Game." It is no coincidence that this surge in popularity of professional football came during a postwar reckoning of the blurring of the roles of men and women, and during a prosperous period when American society became increasingly conformist, yet worried about a physical decline. President-elect John F. Kennedy wrote in *Sports Illustrated* that the "age of leisure and abundance" had created "The Soft American." *Esquire* published an essay during this period titled "The Crisis of American Masculinity." The solution to this crisis, of course, was more football. Even the most genteel American thinkers realized football was on its path to becoming known as a sport of selflessness and sacrifice, of teamwork and of real American men, the true American sport.

"The rise of pro football and relative decline in the popularity of Major League Baseball seems more momentous, a demarcation between past and present, not merely in sports but in the culture itself," MacCambridge writes. "This is true for several reasons, among them the speed with which pro football surpassed baseball, and the fact that well into the 1950s, so few people saw it coming . . . 'Whoever wants to know the heart and mind of America had better know baseball,' wrote [French-American historian] Jacques Barzun in 1954 . . . But in the span of two generations in postwar America, pro football became a truer and more vivid reflection of the American preoccupations with power and passion, technology and teamwork, than any other sporting institution in the country."

Football would continue to rise. A competing league, the American Football League, was founded in 1959, the year after the landmark Colts-Giants game. In 1961, the NFL signed its first national television contract. Soon, the leagues merged, which led to the first Super Bowl in 1967. NFL Commissioner Pete Rozelle turned football into a sport with broad middle-class appeal. Nineteen of the twenty most-watched American television programs ever are football games. (The other had an even more direct tie to violence and to the military: the series finale of *M*A*S*H*.)

Over the next few decades, football became an American staple. In a world that seemed to be simultaneously shrinking and expanding through new technology and media, through political upheaval and international migration, football was something Americans could count on as a simple morality play: one hundred yards from end zone to end zone, four downs to get ten yards, eleven men per side, may the best man win. It became a sport that helped unify a balkanizing nation. From the coasts to the landlocked plains, football captured the imagination of fans and businessmen and sportswriters alike, so it's only natural that the sport spread into families' backyards. In Indianola, Iowa, the Easter family looked at football as a sport of truth and beauty, a game whose physical and mental challenges constituted a rite of passage from boyhood into manhood. Zac Easter looked at football as a compulsory joy. Quite simply, football was something that Easter men did: Easter men like his father, the former Division I scholarship player who became a college and high school coach. Easter men like his older brother, who also got a college scholarship to play football. Even Easter men like his younger brother, who never really took to the sport but who felt compelled to play for the high school team anyway. To Zac, football was far more than just some game you watched on Saturdays (the Iowa Hawkeyes) and Sundays (the Green Bay Packers). Football was a test of your manhood. Don't play football and you're not a man. Football was looking at the pain intrinsic in the sport as a gift, something worth fighting through to build one's character. Like Vince Lombardi had said, "The good Lord gave you a body that can stand most anything. It's your mind you have to convince."

Years later, even as Zac Easter's mind was breaking apart, he wrote words that would have made Lombardi proud: "I remember being one of the hardest hitting linebackers ever since I started . . . I learned around this age that if I used my head as a weapon and literally put my head down on every play up until the last play I ever played. I was always shorter than a lot of other players and learned to put my head down so I could have the edge and win every battle. Not only that, but I liked the attention I got from the coaches and other players."

At the time, that way of thinking still seemed admirable.

BEFORE ZAC WAS born, Myles Sr. took a job as defensive coordinator at Simpson College, a Division III school in Indianola. He never *made* his boys play football—it was more like it was just assumed. "I loved football," he said. "I was getting to the point where I loved it more than the kids did back in high school." Not that the boys didn't love it, too. As little kids, they'd come to Myles's practice every day and hang off to the side with the kickers. By third grade, Zac was playing full-contact football in helmet and pads, like most other boys in his town.

His dad's expectations and his older brother's example—the "Easter mentality," as people called it in Indianola—were a lot for young Zac to live up to. "I was tired of teachers and even Principal Monroe comparing me to my brother and asking me why I wasn't as good of a student as my older brother," Zac wrote. "I guess I got to the point then where I just didn't care and realized the only way to [feel] adequate to fill the Easter family shoes was to play football."

To his teammates and friends, who didn't see the mental struggles that were covered up by Zac's hard-ass attitude, Zac became

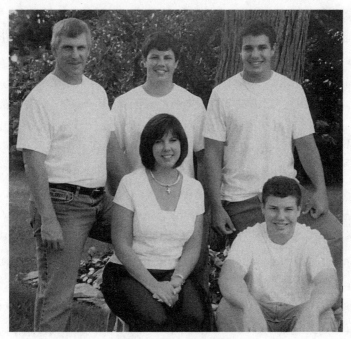

The Easter family:
(front row, left to right) Brenda and Levi.
(back row, left to right) Myles Sr., Zac, Myles II.

a heroic sort of figure. "You could ask any of our friends who was the biggest prick on the field, and it was Zac," Nick Haworth, one of Zac's best friends since childhood who played football with him through high school, said admiringly. "When you're playing like a prick, you're getting after it, and that's what Zac did. He didn't take shit from anybody. And he hit *hard*. And Zac, that sonofabitch, when he hit, he used his head. He wanted to be tough, man."

"I won't lie," Zac wrote. "I look back now and always felt like I had something to prove to my dad and trying to fill my older brothers football shoes."

He added, "I'm sure [my dad] loves me but he's always had a hard time showing it. I feel like all my concussions were for him in the first place because I just wanted to impress him and feel tough."

Zac wasn't born with what he needed to become a football star, so in high school he secretly began taking prohormones, a steroid-like supplement banned in many sports. Zac's father didn't know about the supplements. But he noticed Zac, who'd always been a little chubby, getting into phenomenal shape. Myles Sr. and his boys would sometimes grab a few Coors Lights and go down to the basement for bench press contests. Before those sessions, Myles Sr. always told Zac that he'd bench press fifty pounds more than him. One day when Zac was in high school, he bench pressed 285 pounds of metal. "OK," his father said, "I can beat that." Myles Sr. was working his way up in weight when he pushed 315 pounds of metal off his chest and . . . *Pop!* He tore a pectoral muscle.

One way Zac asserted himself against his father and older brother was by defecting from the family's NFL team, the Minnesota Vikings, to the Green Bay Packers. It was Zac's mischievous streak at work. While Myles II sat alongside his father in Vikings purple-and-gold, Zac shouted, "Go, Pack, go!" He relished the opportunity to rib his older brother and dad. Zac loved Brett Favre—he had the same swagger as Favre, the same gunslinger mentality, the same imperviousness to pain—and his dad finally relented and got him a Packers jersey emblazoned with Favre's number: 4. Favre might have been a quarterback and Zac a fullback/linebacker, positions that require different mentalities, but Favre's throw-caution-to-the-wind approach and his much-admired ability to play through pain seemed heroic to Zac. Myles II might have been taller and faster than his brother, talented enough to earn a college football scholarship and a spot in his high school's sports hall of fame, but Zac was always the toughest dude on the field. "He was out there to fuck people up," said Myles II. "He was there to do some damage."

TWO

The Ancestors

IN THE SPRING of 1854, Jacob Stickler, a fifty-three-year-old man of German descent—the great-great-great-great-grandfather of Zac Easter—decided to quit his backbreaking work in the Pennsylvania coal mines and head west. Like anyone willing to brave the dangers and uncertainties of America's frontier, Stickler was in search of a new beginning. He left his wife and daughter behind, hitched the horses to his wagon, and headed toward the same place where so many other Pennsylvania coal miners were going: to the gently rolling hills of Iowa, a haven of rich, black, sandy soil and miles upon miles of prairie land ripe for grazing. The land was plentiful, and, through the Manifest Destiny way of thinking that led white men to settle on land long occupied by Native Americans, the land was also his for the taking. At the time of Stickler's trip toward the frontier, the eastern migration to Iowa was at its height. Iowa's population in 1840 was only about forty-three thousand people, or less than one person per square mile statewide. A decade later, after Iowa had been admitted as the twenty-ninth state in the Union, its population had nearly quintupled, to nearly two hundred thousand people. Those people's fortunes rested on living off the land, and in time, the settlers would turn Iowa into one of America's most productive agricultural areas, the breadbasket of a booming nation.

If the final leg of Stickler's trip was anything like that of his fellow travelers, it could not have been particularly pleasant. Roaming the Iowa prairies at the time were not only plenty of buffalo and deer that could provide sustenance for an able hunter but also animals that presented danger: wolves and badgers, wildcats and rattlesnakes. Plagues of Rocky Mountain locusts—settlers derisively referred to them as grasshoppers—would occasionally wipe out the sun while devouring everything from cropland to clothing right off people's backs.

Though his new home was a grueling thousand-mile trip from his old home, what Stickler would find when he arrived in Iowa was both comfortably familiar and thrillingly foreign. Some migrants referred to Iowa and its agricultural bounty as the El Dorado of that time, so valued was that black gold; heading to Iowa was for these frontiersmen like the Spanish conquistadors and other European explorers searching for that mythical lost city of gold. Yet Iowa was also a place that was strikingly similar to the home Stickler had known back East, at least in terms of the white people who lived there. As a fellow Iowa settler wrote in a letter at the time: "We have a good and we think nice country, and good society, the majority being Pennsylvanians."

Stickler homesteaded 240 acres of land, hills and timber and prairie, where muddy eroding cliffs descended to the meandering North River and Howerdon Creek. It was not far south of Des Moines, which in 1857 would be named the capital of the new state. No white man had lived on this land before, though it had been home to generations of Native Americans. A nearby village for the Sac and Fox tribes had been abandoned only a decade before Stickler staked his claim to the land. For the next 150 years, Jacob Stickler and his descendants would occasionally unearth an

old arrowhead or tomahawk blade while they were tending the
fields or walking the timber. The closest hub of settlers' civilization
was a recently plotted town called Winterset a few miles away. The
place was originally going to be called Summerset; an unseasonable
cold spell during the summer when settlers were debating what to
call their new home caused them to change their minds. Stickler's
first year there could not have been easy. He spent that first winter
holed up in the same covered wagon in which he'd made the long
journey. His wife, Rachel, and their only child, a grown daughter
named Diana, came later, after that long winter.

Diana was married to a man named William Miner Ford, a
West Virginian by birth who'd also worked in the Pennsylvania
coal mines. It was the two of them who established the family
farm in 1855 on the land Jacob Stickler had settled on the year
before. These were heady times in Iowa—the state's population
had more than doubled in the five years since the 1850 census. The
Fords had four children, all born in Iowa. The second-youngest,
Emma, who was born just as the Civil War was beginning, married
a man named Josiah Easter a few days after Christmas in 1879,
when both were still teenagers. It was around this time when Iowa
youths started playing the new, tough-minded sport of American
football, on fields that ranged from stockyards to fairgrounds to
pastures. Josiah took over the family farm in 1895 after his father-
in-law passed away. For generations that followed, the family grew
the same crops and raised the same animals that most Iowans
did: corn and soybeans, cattle and hogs and chickens, and always
supplemented by an enormous garden. Josiah and Emma had ten
children. The youngest was born in 1906, a boy named William
Ford Easter. The same country doctor who delivered William Ford
Easter would, the very next year, deliver another baby in town who

would come to define a generation of American manhood: Marion Robert Morrison, who later changed his name to John Wayne.

A childhood spent working and romping the family's acreage shaped William Ford Easter, just as it would shape generations of Easter men after him—especially his great-grandson Zac. As a boy, William would join his father in riding through the family's timber in a horse-drawn wagon, the two of them wielding axes to cut down trees for firewood. Sometimes, as Josiah steered the wagon on the edge of their property along an old buggy trail that stretched all the way to Winterset, the horses would suddenly stop. The horses wouldn't move another inch, acting nervous and fidgety. The boy would be scared, but his dad would hop down from the wagon, aim his double-barreled shotgun at the tall grass, and blast to smithereens the rattlesnake that was agitating his horses. The lesson to his son was clear, and the lesson would be passed on from each generation of this family just as it had been since Jacob Stickler homesteaded here: The meek would not inherit this slice of the earth. Life here was for men who were tough and fearless.

William Ford Easter had a bit of a wild streak when he was younger, according to family lore. Being tough and fearless was one thing; being reckless and disrespectful was quite another. Once, as a teenager, William mounted one of the horses from the barn, took it into town, and raced it on the downtown streets. That infuriated his no-nonsense father, Josiah, so much that William would still be telling that story a half century later. But eventually, he settled into the life that was expected of him, a hardworking life on the farm, growing crops and raising animals. Occasionally, he'd still feed those wild urges of his earlier years, like when he went up in a World War I–era open-cockpit biplane one winter day with his brother, flew low over the farm and aimed his 12-gauge shotgun at the foxes that had been killing his farm animals. He shot three of them.

Easter men have never relied on other people to fix their problems. Since their forebears first began to tame their rough, hilly patch of land in Iowa, they have always taken pride in handling challenges on their own. When the family transitioned from farming with horses to using modern farm machinery around the time of World War II, doing so came with an added responsibility for William Ford Easter, as well as an added joy. He loved it when farm machinery broke down because that meant he got to repair it. One year, he bought two used, nonfunctioning combines. He spent the entire winter fusing the parts of those two combines into one working machine. To make ends meet, he got a job managing the Ford garage in nearby Saint Charles. He adored the Ford Model T, the first mass-produced car that had been introduced to the American public when he was two years old. When he bought one of those Model Ts brand-new, his father told him he was wasting his money on such a fancy car. A couple of years later, he sold it—and he'd taken such good care of it that he recouped what he'd paid for it.

William Ford Easter married a woman named Blanche Kuntz, and together they weathered the Depression and the Dust Bowl the only way they knew how: By being frugal, by never buying anything they didn't need, and by heading to the nearby country church down the rocky road, where William sang a sonorous tenor in the choir as they prayed for God's help in taming this unpredictable land. During the bruising winters, the Easters heated only one room of the house at a time with fuel they'd cut from the family's timber, shutting the rest of the doors of the house to trap the heat in that one room. They never took on debt, and after the banks went bust, they had piles of cash savings stuffed around their house. Perhaps because of the economic struggles of the time and how they affected child-rearing, they only had one child, William Kuntz Easter: "Willie K," Zac Easter's grandfather.

Willie K was born in the early 1930s, as the Dust Bowl raged throughout the American plains. It was during those years that the farm was at its lowest point. One growing season, it produced exactly one bushel of rye grass: nothing more, the rest of the farm just dirt and dust. Around that time, William Ford Easter decided he'd get on a horse and ride it 370 miles east to Chicago, where he planned to march into a bank and cash in his cash-value life insurance policy to scrape together more money. When he got to Chicago, though, the life insurance company had gone belly-up. From that day on, William said life insurance was "all a bunch of bullshit." That story became legend in the Easter family, and it enshrined their frugal ways. It wasn't until Willie K was a high school senior that the family got electricity in their farmhouse, and even then, they didn't overuse what they saw as a luxury. Until the day William Ford Easter died in 1995, he'd never put more than one light bulb in a light fixture that had space for six. But even as the family scratched out a living throughout the Depression, there was always a pride in doing things their own way, and a pride in being a part of an America that had only itself to rely on.

One of Willie K's most distinct memories from his childhood was during World War II, when female fighter pilots—the Women Airforce Service Pilots—would fly low over the farm, transporting military bombers from one coast to the other. Moments like that connected this family to the great national pride that stemmed from conquering the Nazis in World War II. And for a family like

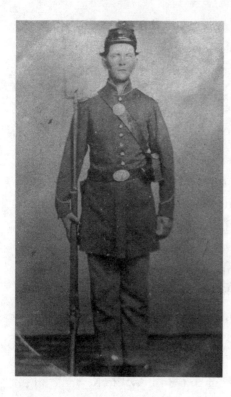

Zac's great-great-great-grandfather, William C. Easter, fought with the 30th Iowa Volunteer Infantry Regiment during the Civil War.

the Easters—whose military service stretched from the great-great-great-grandfather who was shot in the leg during the first charge at the Battle of Vicksburg on July 4, 1863, all the way to Zac, who went through army boot camp and had dreams of becoming an Army Ranger—words about patriotism were more than just empty platitudes.

Willie K, who served in the army and the air force in the period between the Korean War and the Vietnam War, married a local woman named Meredith Young. They had met in their high school band, where he played saxophone and she played oboe and was the drum majorette. Her family, which had been in Iowa for just as long as his family had, owned the hardware store near Winterset's town square—it's still owned and operated by her descendants today. In 1870, her family had built the Cutler-Donahoe Covered Bridge in Winterset, one of the six covered bridges that have given Madison County its international renown. Her family also owned the grain elevator in town. The marriage was a union of two farming families that had lived within a few miles of each other for five generations, and it resulted in three children: Chuck, who would eventually take over the family farm; Melody, who would become close childhood friends with Brenda Nicholson, who lived in the town of Winterset; and the oldest, Myles, who would eventually marry Brenda and have three sons with her. Myles and Brenda named their middle boy Zachary Joseph Easter.

To say that Zac Easter's vision of what defined a true American man can be directly traced to his father and his father's strenuous childhood on the family farm is plainly true, but it understates how deep this family's roots run in the tough, macho, survivalist ethic of Midwest farming life. After seven generations living on what would eventually become 543 acres of Easter family farmland and timber, the Easter mentality became something that was virtually ingrained in the family's DNA. By the twenty-first century, this tough ethos led Easter men not to the feedlot or the grain bin but instead to the high school football field in neighboring Indianola. The Easter mentality now meant something more singular and narrow: the toughness and stoicism and self-sacrifice that created the best football players, the sport that has come to represent the most extreme possibilities of the male body as well as the male mind.

OVER THE PAST several years, as the connection between football and brain injuries has become ever more clear, the NFL's marketing effort has taken on a nostalgic tinge. Instead of directly confronting

American families' fear of the toll football takes on those who play it, the NFL instead has reminded Americans that football is more than just a sport. It's also a central part of family life in America. In 2012, former NFL linebacker Junior Seau's suicide marked an inflection point in the American conversation about head injuries in football. The year after Seau's suicide, the NFL's league-wide marketing slogan became "Together We Make Football." The campaign focused on the lifelong relationships and bonds that are forged and fostered through the sport. A couple of years later, the league's marketing campaign was "Football Is Family." It is not a coincidence that in the midst of the sport's biggest existential crisis in a century—since Teddy Roosevelt gathered football leaders and university leaders to clean up the ultraviolent, dangerous sport—the NFL sought to remind Americans that many of their most cherished relationships are tied up in football.

Much of the story of the relationship between American fathers and sons can be told through sports, often through football, the most American and most manly of sports. When the future of football is debated in the public sphere, the pro-football argument frequently reverts to the nostalgia of childhood: the memories of the thrill of Friday night lights, or of spending fall weekends in front of the television with Dad and Grandpa, or of the way August two-a-day practices were the greatest of lessons in how to become a man. The sport has been lauded as the best sport to make a great man, and the best sport to make a great nation.

The roots of America's most popular, most lucrative, most addictive sport can be traced back to an almost medieval, primal mentality that became an inexorable part of American history and its obsession with military power and Manifest Destiny. As Senator Henry Cabot Lodge of Massachusetts put it about football more than a century ago: "The injuries incurred on the playing-field are part of the price which the English-speaking race has paid for being world-conquerors."

The sport's roots go far deeper than that 1869 Rutgers–College of New Jersey game, and much further back in history. There's evidence of similar games being played throughout the millennia. More than two thousand years ago, the Chinese were playing a game called *cuju*, or "kickball," and evidence of football's other ancestors can be found in ancient Greece, Rome, and Japan. But the most direct antecedent for American football dates to England more than five hundred years ago. Rugby is football's uncle, and rugby itself had derived from the sport Americans know as soccer—or, well, "football," as people in the Old Country began calling it because the sport was played on foot instead of on horseback. The roots of Old World football can be traced back to England's medieval period. The earliest versions of the sport, as it were, were played on Sundays and on Shrove Tuesday each year as battles between young peasant men of competing villages. The young men of one team kicked a ball, which was either a bull's head or an animal bladder, from their village to the rival village. There were barely any rules.

Even from its earliest days, people worried about the sport's violent nature. In 1531, as Henry VIII ruled over England, the English statesman Sir Thomas Elyot called football "nothynge but beastlye furie and exstreme violence . . . malice and rancor do remain with they that be wounded." This primitive game eventually morphed into the sport Americans know as soccer, though not without controversy. Major injuries and deaths occurred frequently during the early versions of this sport. Oxford and Cambridge both banned it for a time. Then came a tweak that would eventually lead toward

American football. "A deviant form of the game ensued in 1823 when William Webb Ellis, a student at the Rugby School in England, allegedly picked up the ball and ran with it," Gerald R. Gems, a sports historian, wrote in his book, *For Pride, Profit and Patriarchy: Football and the Incorporation of American Cultural Values*.

The nineteenth century heralded the beginning of modern sports—*modern* meaning a set of static rules were written down and a referee was instituted to ensure people followed those rules. The development of soccer and rugby in England came during a time of great change during and after the Industrial Revolution, as country folk moved into cities, as police forces were developed, and as people's lives underwent greater regulation in these urbanized societies than they'd ever experienced before. Sport afforded urban dwellers an outlet as well as a proving ground.

In America, the "sport" of football began as really nothing more than controlled riots on college campuses: a hazing ritual. In the early to middle 1800s, upperclassmen rushed through college campuses en masse with the intent of harming the freshmen. Harvard and Yale both banned the game in 1860, which also happened to be the same year that secondary schools on the East Coast first started playing football. The first national rules convention took place in 1873. Another rules convention, in 1880, helped form the version of the sport we know today; that's when Walter Camp, "the Father of American Football," introduced the concept of a line of scrimmage. This differentiated the organized nature of American football from the more chaotic nature of rugby. While rugby had a mass *scrummage* after every tackle, the line of *scrimmage* allowed one team to retain possession of the ball for a period of time instead of having to fight for it after every play.

This also made the sport more like modern warfare, which created the illusion of a welcome antidote to what society worried was an increasingly emasculated American male. In the period after the Civil War, when the American sport of football first took hold, more Americans moved to cities. That meant men no longer had to meet the everyday rigors of living off the land to provide for their families. Traditional masculine traits seemed less important in these urban settings, where people now toiled behind desks. That masculine anxiety was only heightened by the increasing calls for women's suffrage, and by the expanding role of women in the working life. In 1870, 21 percent of college students were women. Ten years later, that grew to almost 36 percent; by 1920, it was more than 47 percent. In 1880, there were only thirty-two women lawyers in all of America; by 1910, there were 1,341. There were five times as many female doctors in America in 1910 as there were in 1880.

The rapidity of the cultural shift was acute. A fear of an increasingly feminized American culture provoked a masculine backlash that took many forms: from aggressive foreign policy to medicines that purported to boost manliness and vitality, from the sudden booms in bodybuilding and Western fiction to the increasing popularity of the "manly sport" of football. American men felt diminished during this period, and football offered a controlled setting in which they could prove their manhood in the face of physical danger. In the same tradition as fighting competitions between knights in the Middle Ages, football became the ultimate public display of masculinity.

On top of that, the peaceful period after the Civil War meant American men could no longer prove their mettle through battlefield exploits. Football, then, became "surrogate war," in the words of several historians, a way to gain the mentality forged in wartime while participating in an activity that didn't induce mass casualties. The idea of a team retaining possession of the ball for a set period of "downs"—proposed by Walter Camp—required more strategic maneuvers on the part of players and coaches: plays that were planned in advance, specific roles for each position, and responsibilities for all players that required working together as a single unit. This new sport was billed as a competition of military preparedness— "mimic battlefield," as one early proponent of football called the sport—as well as a training ground for future corporate leaders. "If ever a sport offered inducements to the man of executive ability, to the man who can plan, foresee and manage," wrote Camp, "it is certainly the modern American football."

"As the United States began to emerge as a world power," sports historian Gerald R. Gems wrote, "football provided significant messages to both American and foreign onlookers. The game elicited comparisons with the battlefield where 'two armies are managed on military principles . . . ,' and the 'American' competition was judged 'one of the most scientific of outdoor games . . . where players worked with 'clock-work precision.' In the aggressive, competitive, industrial modern world, football served as a training ground." The football field became a training ground for both generals and executives. It is not too much of a stretch to think of football as the perfect place of indoctrination for the uniquely American ethos of Manifest Destiny—the nation's inevitable expansion throughout the continent—and to the imperialistic mindset America took on in the twentieth century. At its most elemental, football is a series of violent marches into an enemy's territory, where one team gains land at the expense of the other team. At the time of football's rise, Americans certainly understood those analogies to infantry warfare, where one team tries to find the greatest weakness in the other team's line, and then attacks.

WHEN ZAC WAS five years old, his father took him to hunt pheasant for the first time. Myles Sr. was five when his own father first took him to hunt pheasant. The outing with Zac was muddy and cold. They were in the back corner of a field, as far away as possible from the farmhouse, when Zac did what most five-year-olds would do: He started whining.

"Dad, carry me!" he whined. "I can't walk anymore!"

"I ain't carrying your ass," Myles replied. "You're hunting."

It was an early lesson in being a man.

After a few minutes, Zac piped up again.

"Dad, I think I'm going to die," he moaned.

"Well, OK—well then, die," his dad replied. "The crows and buzzards will eat you. We'll be OK."

All of a sudden, Zac got a surge of energy. He made it through the rest of the hunt. His father told him afterward that he was proud of him. The lesson stuck, and so did Zac's love of hunting, a real man's hobby if there ever was one. When each of his sons turned eleven years old, Myles would take him on his first deer hunt with the boy actually carrying a gun. "It was kind of like Christmas, all the anticipation," Brenda Easter said. "The boys would get so excited. All three of them couldn't wait." By the time they were eleven, they knew not to complain while they were out hunting with their dad.

This moment for each of them marked the seeds of the tough, stoic mentality being passed from father to son. What real men do is battle through the pain. They certainly don't whine about it. But the Easter boys' childhood was not without love. Far from it. It's just that this sort of love was a love of a hardscrabble man whose family had worked the land for six generations, and who disdained the modern-day softening of society, with men who were supposed to be in touch with their feelings and with boys who could no longer be boys. "Today, you can't have the same childhood that I had," Myles Easter said. But he tried to instill in his boys the same ethic that came out of his own upbringing, these modern ways be damned.

Astute observers could see a lot of Zac's great-grandpa, William Ford Easter—the one who took joyrides on the family's horses and flew the biplane low over the fields while hunting foxes—in the little boy: the sweet, curious kid who always wanted to learn how things worked and how he could fix them but also had a devious streak that made him determined to break stuff. Seven-year-old Zac disassembling a Tonka truck to see how it worked sounds just like William Ford Easter deconstructing and then reassembling those old combines. Like his great-grandpa, Zac had a mischievous streak that bedeviled his parents. In the woods with his brothers, Zac would toss an M-80 firecracker down a hole to scare out a snake or two. If the boys were lucky enough to capture a snake, they'd stuff another M-80 down its throat and blow its head off. Zac was fearless, confident that he could push his body to its outermost limits—invincible.

THREE

The Father

ON A CHILLY spring day not too long ago, I stood with Myles Easter Sr. in the family's kitchen as he wondered how everything had gone so wrong. Around his neck he wore a chain with a metal pendant that was a reproduction of Zac's thumbprint. He knew Zac was as in love with football's violence as he was, and he was still proud of Zac's toughness, in spite of everything. Myles took a heavy breath, then he spoke, his voice a stew of pride and guilt: "He was my type of guy." The natural human reaction when tragedy strikes is to look inward, to examine your own role, to wonder if you could have prevented it somehow. What if you'd turned left instead of right? What if you'd said something encouraging to a loved one when he was feeling at his lowest? What if Zac had never played football, had never ruined his brain?

What if?

But Myles Easter Sr. is a man's man, not prone to hours of self-reflection or weekly appointments with a psychotherapist. As America's coasts and metropolises become stereotypical havens for sensitive hipsters, the old-school tough-it-out archetype of the American male lives on in the places in between, perhaps nowhere more saliently than in small towns and rural areas throughout the Midwest. After his middle son's suicide, Myles's wife suggested they and their sons, Myles II and Levi, all go to counseling. "I don't need that shit" was his response.

Myles Easter was born in 1961, the year after Frank Gifford suffered one of the most famous on-field concussions in NFL history, the year the Minnesota Vikings became the fourteenth NFL team, and the year that an influential medical report sparked a debate on whether the newfangled plastic helmets actually were more effective that the old leather ones. The oldest of three children, he was raised on that same land that had been homesteaded by his great-great-great-grandfather more than a century before. Myles's father worked the farm; his mother cooked three meals a day, raised the children, and taught private music lessons to help make ends meet.

There were a few constants in Myles's early life: farm animals, dogs, guns, and football. The animals around the farm were his daily company, from the good animals, like the hogs that made the family money, to the bad animals, like the foxes and snakes that were forever menaces. Life lived in conjunction with domesticated animals and in competition with wild animals brought an element of unpredictability and stoicism to Myles' childhood. A rat bit him at age five, and for the next sixteen days straight, he had to get a daily rabies shot in his stomach. Moments like this bred a no-complaints sense of toughness from a young age. Early each morning, he was outside with his dad, doing farm chores, feeding and watering the hogs that roamed the timber. In winter, they pulled the hogs out of the timber and grazed them in the field, where the hogs would devour corn left over from the harvest. Getting the hogs out of the timber was the most dangerous part. "You pull up to the gate, you better be ready," Myles recalled. "We got food, and those hogs are running! They're all hauling ass, sprinting at your ass, and they're grunting: 'WOOF! WOOF!' I'm opening the gate, my dad's driving in fast, and then I gotta shut the gate fast so they don't get out."

When Myles was five, his father gave him a couple of hogs to tend to on his own. He named them Zebra and Rhino, and eventually sold the pair for sixteen dollars. Raising those hogs helped give Myles the toughness and work ethic to one day become a classic football man. There's something about castrating hogs—heading into the barn early on a cool fall morning, pinning the hog down with your legs, pulling up the hog's back leg as the animal is kicking you and fighting you, and then snipping off its balls and feeding them to the dogs—that feels like a perverse sort of training for football.

Another constant throughout Myles's childhood: dogs. The dogs he had were always beagles or coonhounds, and he named almost all of them Skippy. The reason he had so many different dogs during his childhood? They kept getting run over. It was one of Myles's early lessons about the fragility of life. When Myles was in eighth grade, an older local boy in a truck ran over Skippy. Instead of expressing sorrow for killing the coonhound, the boy just laughed. Some years later, when Myles was in college, he saw that same driver who'd killed his dog. "Remember me?" Myles asked his old nemesis. Then, Myles punched him in the mouth.

Another constant was guns. Yes, the guns were for utility, for killing the rattlesnakes and foxes that menaced their farm animals, and for hunting the deer and pheasant that were in abundance on the family's land. But the guns were also for entertainment. Myles was a quiet and serious boy. Most of his childhood joy involved himself, his dog, and his gun. For Myles's ninth birthday, his dad got him a BB gun. "That's all I did, every day, shooting that BB gun," Myles recalled. "Shooting birds, sparrows. I shot a screech owl one time out in the barn. Shot a rabbit one time with it. At night, I'd go out to the barn with my headlamp on. We'd shoot twenty sparrows or starlings a night. The cats and dogs would go out and eat them." The summer before he turned thirteen, he walked the bean fields all summer and pulled weeds, saving up fifty dollars. With that he bought a big bluetick coonhound named Duke.

A final constant in Myles's childhood: football. One of the oldest black-and-white photographs from his childhood shows him dressed up in a football uniform as a toddler. "I loved football right out of the gate," he recalls. Starting when Myles was three, Grandpa Easter would pick up him and his father on fall Friday evenings, and they would drive to Winterset, meet up with Myles's other grandfather, and walk to the high school to cheer on the local football team. Even at age four or five, Myles was transfixed by the spectacle, the strategy, and the savagery—the big hits on the field that got the loudest shouts from the crowd, and that seemed to young Myles to define what it meant to be a real man. On other nights, Myles would go to his maternal grandparents' house, and they'd listen on the radio to football games from the big Catholic high school in Des Moines. It's a scene that would repeat when Myles had grown boys of his own, when he and Zac and Myles II and Levi would stand outside the truck on a Friday night, drink beers, and listen to high school games on the truck's radio.

As a kid, Myles Sr. also went to Iowa State games seventy miles away in Ames with his grandfathers. When Iowa State played a small private school in Des Moines called Drake University, Myles turned to his father and said, "I want to play for Drake." He liked the uniforms. In high school, Myles played strong safety, and he loved to hit people—hard. His favorite team was the Minnesota Vikings, a bruising crew whose defensive line became known as the Purple People Eaters. But his favorite player didn't play for the Vikings. He played for the Oakland Raiders. It was Jack Tatum, the hardest-hitting safety of his time, nicknamed "the Assassin." Tatum is remembered for paralyzing an opponent with a big hit during a preseason game. Myles channeled that on the field. He still beams when talking about those perfect hits, the ones that felt pure and true and utterly destructive. "I had a few of those hits where you really don't feel it because you smoked the guy so bad," Myles recalled of his own playing career, which progressed from Winterset High School to Drake University, just as he'd predicted as a kid. "I was always hungry for those. I was a Vikings fan, but Jack Tatum *killed* people. He blew people up. And that's what I liked about football."

Myles Easter paused after he told me this. It had been four decades since Tatum's big hit paralyzed wide receiver Darryl Stingley, sixteen years since Dr. Bennet Omalu performed the autopsy of NFL Hall of Famer Mike Webster and found anomalies in his brain, six years since NFL star Junior Seau pointed a shotgun at his own chest and killed himself at age forty-three, and not even three years since his own son Zac had committed suicide at twenty-four—after only playing football through high school.

He sighed. Part of him still looked at the biggest of football hits as one of the great markers of real manhood; you don't just erase that way of thinking after it had been etched into your brain for a half century. "You didn't know people were getting hurt that bad," he said, almost by way of apology. "That was the innocence of football when I was younger."

Today, his feelings on football are nuanced and complex. He hates what the sport had done to his son, yet like so many millions of Americans, he still loves football. He spends Sundays in the fall watching his Vikings. He even took over Zac's fantasy football team after his death. He still finds himself addicted to the sport's cathartic form of violence—at least the violence that the sport *used* to have. But increasingly, as the concussion crisis has spurred a safety revolution in football, and as rule changes have "sissified" the game—Myles's word—the sport of today does not resemble the sport he grew up loving. As he looks at the current style of football, a style that increasingly favors finesse and speed over hard hits and an old-school sense of manliness, he hates this version of the sport in spite of himself. This isn't *real* football. The sport has become safer than even a few years ago, certainly, as fears of an epidemic of head injuries had spurred the NFL, colleges, high schools, and youth leagues to try to take the head out of the game. Myles realizes this is a very good thing, both for the football players as well as for the survival of the sport. But the game at times appears unrecognizable when compared with the sport he revered during his childhood.

"I don't even like watching football anymore," Myles Easter said with a shrug.

His reasoning is not so much because the sport had contributed to the death of his son, and not so much because the sport was going through this existential crisis as fans and parents grappled with how much violence was an acceptable amount of violence. His feelings on football have waned because of this: "It's just gotten to be a track meet."

In Myles Easter's mind, it's not that there is too much violence in football these days. It's that there isn't enough.

MYLES EASTER TEACHING his three sons the sport of football can be viewed two ways. On the simplest level, it's one man who enjoyed a game and shared that game with his boys. No different than a father passing on to his children a love of chess, or wood-working, or comic books. But Myles as his sons' first football coach can take on a deeper, almost anthropological aspect: A tribal elder passes on the ideas of violence to the younger men of his tribe, a lifelong lesson in the skills of warfare that are intended to protect and expand their society. That's what you hear when Myles Sr. talks about his own football career, a joyful worship of the sport's violent side: "I just wanted to knock the fuck out of somebody," he said. His favorite teams were what he now looks at as old-school teams, before there were newfangled pass-happy spread offenses (he prefers three yards and a cloud of dust) and rules that protect and even coddle the quarterbacks (rules that he believes softens the game). Football and violence are part of the recipe to create a man.

Of course, training young men for the battlefield, whether through actual military training or through the "surrogate war" that is football, has also meant coarsening them to violence. Not all of America has been on board for that. Football's history has been marked by a push-pull between two forces in society: the motherly concern that football's violence goes too far versus the feeling of the red-blooded American male that sometimes football's violence isn't just acceptable but *necessary*. The game encouraged violence among its players and bloodlust among the increasing numbers of spectators who came to watch. A new rules convention in 1883 allowed for any manner of violence: "to hack, throttle, butt, trip up, tackle below the hips, or strike an opponent with closed fist three times before he was sent from the field." A downed ball carrier might keep crawling forward, fighting for every inch as tacklers piled on top of him and kneed him and kicked him until he verbally admitted defeat.

An 1888 *New York Times* story about a Yale–College of New Jersey game detailed the game's brutality: "The favorite methods of damaging an opponent were to stamp on his feet, to kick his shins, to give him a dainty upper cut, and to gouge his face in tackling . . . He gets on his feet again, limps around a little, gathers his wandering wits and is as eager for the fray as ever." This violence was both accepted as part of the nature of the game as well as glorified as what made the game great. There was beauty amidst the game's brutality, and the game's brutality made that beauty stand out even more. By 1890, the beauty and brutality had spread to Iowa when high schools in the Hawkeye State started playing organized football.

But the point of football was never the beauty; the point was battling through the brutality. Men who could withstand this level of violence were thought of as better men. A Harvard coach during the late 1800s refused to allow on his field doctors, medicine, or even timeouts, fearing that any of those would turn his players into "babies." A popular song from the 1890s about players preparing for a game went like this:

> Just bring along the ambulance,
> And call the Red Cross nurse,
> Then ring the undertaker up,
> And make him bring a hearse;
> Have all the surgeons ready there,
> For they'll have work today,
> Oh, can't you see the football teams,
> Are lining up to play.

As some deified football's violence, others pushed back against it. There have been calls to ban the sport since its inception, and proponents of football have always had to seek that middle ground—to find a level of danger that was still aggressive and manly while also being acceptable to civilized people who watched the sport. When football became a lucrative televised sport, the NFL commissioner wrote into TV contracts that broadcasters couldn't show injuries or fights. "Football's guardians have always tried to walk this absurd line between selling violence and disavowing it," wrote Steve Almond in his book *Against Football: One Fan's Reluctant Manifesto.*

Football's original existential crisis came in the early 1900s. At least forty-five players died nationwide between 1900 and 1905 from injuries suffered during games: internal injuries, broken backs, broken necks and concussions. The *Chicago Tribune* called 1905 the "death harvest" of college football. On the final day of the 1905 season was a marquee game between Harvard and Yale that marked the low point of the sport's early struggles with extreme violence. Francis Burr, a Harvard player, settled under a punt and called for a fair catch. That means he should have been allowed to catch the ball without interference from the opponent. Instead, two Yalies ran straight at him. One punched him in the face and broke his nose. The other "probably delivered a body blow with his feet which knocked Burr 'senseless,'" according to college football historian John Sayle Watterson. It was a brutal play that made headlines nationwide. Burr didn't die, but on that same day, three other football players did die in games: one in New York, one in Indiana, one in Missouri. That added up to at least eighteen fatal injuries during one collegiate football season.

University leaders nationwide began to speak out against football and ban the sport from their campuses. A series of stories in *McClure's* and *Collier's*, two of the most popular magazines of the time, denounced football's brutality and detailed the public outcry against the sport, an outcry led by moralistic educators and religious leaders. (It should be noted that the coach at West Point said in the midst of this controversy that the United States Military Academy at West Point would continue playing football even if other colleges did not.) In Iowa, members of the newly formed Iowa High School Athletic Association banned the sport. Harvard was discussing outlawing the game. A certain resident of the White House read these stories and heard this moral outrage, and he was horrified that his alma mater was considering banning football.

"I emphatically disbelieve in seeing Harvard or any other college turn out molly coddles instead of vigorous men," President Teddy Roosevelt stated. "In any republic, courage is a prime necessity . . . Athletics are good, especially in their rougher forms, because they tend to develop such courage." Roosevelt was a proponent of football's violence—he referred to a victory on the football field as "the prize of death in battle"—but he realized the sport's future depended on making that violence more acceptable, and therefore less savage. (Roosevelt had more personal motivations, too: His eldest son, Ted, had suffered numerous football injuries playing at Groton School and at Harvard, including a broken nose during a Harvard-Yale game.) The president organized a summit at the White House to make the sport less physically dangerous and therefore more palatable to the average American, which led to a special White House commission and testimony before Congress. ("I demand that football change its rules or be abolished," Roosevelt told college officials. "Change the game or forsake it!")

That 1905 summit enacted big changes to make football more recognizable as the sport we know today, establishing a neutral zone at the line of scrimmage, opening up the game to the forward pass, and prohibiting dangerous mass formations like the flying wedge. (The flying wedge was a strategy derived from Napoleon's military tactics.) The summit may have saved American football, and it led to the creation of a national legislative body: the Intercollegiate Athletic Association, which was founded in 1906 and in 1910 became the National Collegiate Athletic Association (NCAA). For a while, it seemed the reforms did make the game safer. The numbers of deaths in college football sank to ten in 1908. That was a temporary salve to the concerns of the antifootball agitators, and Iowa high schools reinstated the sport for the 1909 season.

Despite the concerns, the sport continued its growth; football's ruggedness—its out-and-out embrace of violence—has always been part of its appeal, and perhaps the biggest part. The 1920s was the first decade in which football rivaled baseball as America's most popular sport. While reforms attempted to diminish the most horrific forms of violence, it had by no means disappeared. Another worrisome era in football came in the early 1930s; in 1931, forty-nine players died playing football. All sorts of articles during that period featured titles along the lines of: "Should Your Boy Play Football?" A 1936 issue of *Good Housekeeping* featured a cover illustration of a toddler boy trying on his older brother's football spikes. Inside the magazine was an article, "Death on the Gridiron," that offered a stark warning to parents of football's risks. Even though today's concern over traumatic brain injuries and chronic traumatic encephalopathy has the backing of modern science, these very same (though more visceral) parental concerns about the sport's safety go back more than a century.

At the time, though, most Americans considered these safety risks acceptable because, as the famed sportswriter Grantland Rice wrote, football was a sport that developed "iron in the soul and

steel in the heart." And that's what a nation that often found itself
at war needed to teach its boys, right? Jimmy Conzelman, who
coached the Chicago Cardinals in the 1940s, noted that the mentality football taught was a mentality the nation needed. Especially
during World War II. "They have been taught to build—now they
must learn to destroy," Conzelman said. "Football is the No. 1
medium for attuning a man to body contact and violent physical
shock. It teaches that after all there isn't anything so terrifying
about a punch in the puss."

As the sport matured, regions of this growing nation developed
distinct images for its style of football. Historian Michael Oriard,
who also played several seasons in the NFL, breaks down the
regional football identities this way: The Southwest was defined by
its more speed-oriented passing game. The South was defined by its
"fierce combativeness." And the Midwest, where cold, wet weather
during the fall and winter meant passing was difficult and being
surefooted was valued, had its own version of "rock-'em, sock-
'em power football." The Midwestern style of football—the style
of football that Myles Easter and his three sons adored—seemed
most suited to the type of man Roosevelt hoped America would
breed more of: "the man who is actually in the arena, whose face
is marred by dust, and sweat, and blood."

That type of man also happened to be best suited to the military
life, which may explain why football experienced another era of
growth after World War I. An editorial in the *New York Times* in
1919 explained: "Football owes more to the war in the way of the
spread of the spirit of the game than it does to ten or twenty years of
development in the period before the war." After the war came calls
from the military to expand football. General Leonard Wood said
that America had a preparedness crisis because half of American

men drafted into the military were unfit for duty, and after that came nationwide calls for mandatory athletic programs for youth.

And yet parents continued to ask: Is football safe for my son? Do the benefits outweigh the risk? The role of the football coach began to take on a more paternal dimension. "The football coach bifurcated into this familiar tyrant and an altogether new type: the kindly, nurturing father," Oriard wrote in his magnificent history of media coverage of the sport, *King Football: Sport and Spectacle in the Golden Age of Radio and Newsreels, Movies, and Magazines, the Weekly & the Daily Press*. And this seemed to "have reflected changing ideals of fatherhood and masculinity in the larger culture." Baseball has been sentimentalized in recent decades as the game made for fathers and sons. "You wanna have a catch?" Iowa farmer Ray Kinsella, played by Kevin Costner, asked the ghost of his father in *Field of Dreams*. But baseball is the sport a father turns to when he simply wants to pass time with his son. Football is America's obsession, and points to the more complicated relationships between fathers and sons, "a grittier, more anguished relationship," as Oriard put it. It's the sport that teaches his son about life: that pleasure requires pain, that happiness requires suffering. It is the sport a father turns to when he wants to shape that boy into a man. That framing of football—not just as a hobby or a leisurely pastime but as a sport with undeniable metaphorical parallels to real life—was the reason that by the 1950s, football had become America's most popular sport (despite nineteen football-related deaths in 1959 alone), and that by the twenty-first century, football has become more obsession than game, a vehicle for creating America's alpha males.

"Underlying virtually every narrative of football was the most fundamental issue of all: what it meant to be a 'man,'" Oriard wrote. "While the expanding mass media drove the growth of football's audience, concerns about masculinity were a major factor in making that audience receptive to the game. Brawny and brainy football heroes represented contrasting models of masculinity."

And so it falls right in line with a century and a half of American history that when Myles Easter had his first son, then his second and his third, he yearned for those boys to play the sport he'd played as a boy and still loved as a man. And those boys became burdened with the same burden football players had carried for generations before them: an adult culture that counted on them to win pride for their family and community, to achieve their own and their fathers' ambitions. The way Zac Easter shaped himself into a football player was, in large part, about shaping himself to please his father, and about living up to the exploits of his older brother. Zac the football player was as central a part of his identity as Zac the human being.

His parents knew football carried with it some dangers, though they, like most Americans, had no idea how serious the risk of brain injury was. But they also knew that football created self-assured young men. An Easter man in the twenty-first century no longer had to pack up his life in a covered-wagon migration to show his mettle like Jacob Stickler did a century and a half before. But the Easter mentality still resonated seven generations later, and football was one of its main proving grounds.

MYLES WAS NEARING the final year of his college career as a hard-hitting safety at Drake University when he saw Brenda Nicholson at a New Year's Eve party in 1982. It wasn't the first time they had met. Brenda had been close friends with Myles's little sister, Melody, since middle school. Brenda was a high school cheerleader, but she was also a tomboy. As a little girl, when she had visited

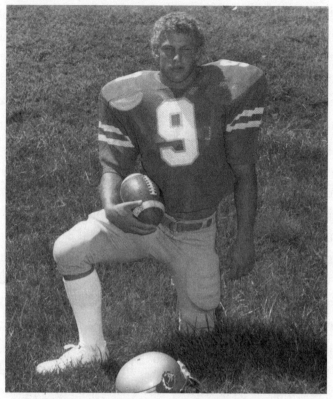

*Myles Sr. was a hard-hitting safety at
Drake University in Des Moines.*

Melody, she'd loved going out to the Easters' land, climbing trees, playing hide-and-seek, catching fireflies and putting them in jars. "It was my heaven," Brenda said. Myles was the big, quiet brother who was always doing farm chores with his dad. They reconnected over keg beer in red Solo cups at that New Year's Eve party. A spark was evident immediately between the big brother and his kid sister's childhood friend. She didn't remember Myles being so incredibly fit back in high school. That's what college football does to a young man. He didn't remember her being so beautiful, with big hair and form-fitting corduroy jeans. They shared their first kiss, and later that night, well after midnight, Myles drove Brenda and two friends back to town. They pulled over to the side of the road for someone to pee. The night was numbingly cold, and the snow was fresh. Brenda hopped out of the truck, and then she slid straight down an embankment, where snow had been piling up. Myles and Brenda both howled with laughter.

The next day, he called her up for pizza, and a relationship quickly blossomed. He was the quieter one, happy to hang with football friends. Brenda was the social butterfly, named "Miss Congeniality" for her high school class (as well as "Best Body"); it was that outgoing, friendly nature that would eventually land her in the ultimate extrovert's job, as the president of the Indianola Chamber of Commerce. Brenda joined the Easter family on long road trips to see Myles's football team play, and even accompanied them when they chartered a plane to fly to a game in Texas. Even though she always cringed at the hardest, scariest hits, Brenda loved watching her big, brawny boyfriend lay into opponents on the field. He was such a fierce competitor that his teammates gave him the nickname "Baby Bull." She wondered why, when he tore up his knee in a game and had to get arthroscopic surgery, he felt football was still worth it, and why he worked so hard to get back on the field. But eventually she came to see his joyful worship of this violent sport as part of what made him such a strong and reliable man.

Brenda fit right in with the Easters: tough and spunky, smart and independent, a country girl through and through. She was always a workout fiend, and later in life, after three kids, would teach intense 5:00 a.m. fitness classes at the local Fusion Fitness. At the same time, she could slam beers right alongside the country

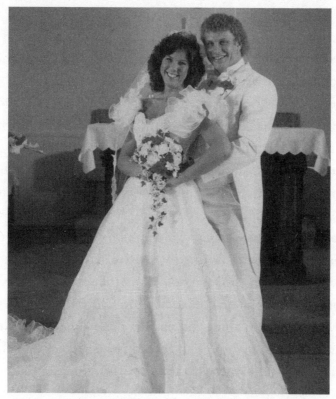

Myles and Brenda reconnected at a party on
New Year's Eve 1982. They married a couple years later.

boys. She was always up for a good time, though her Catholic upbringing generally kept her within the bounds of good taste. (Perhaps the raciest moment of Brenda's high school years was when a group of boys and girls hopped the fence at the community pool and went skinny-dipping.) Brenda was thrilled when Myles invited her to go hunting with him and Duke, the huge bluetick coonhound. They went fishing together, on the farm pond near Myles's parents' house and on the North River in the family's timber. She'd even shoot skeet with her new beau. For Brenda, she simply loved being out in nature with Myles. Within two years, they were married, and a few years later came their first son.

For many people, at this point football would recede into the background: a fun diversion, a way to bond with your sons, nothing more. Not for Myles Easter Sr. When Brenda married him, she also married football. They named their first son Myles II when he was born in 1988, and Myles became known as "Daddy Myles." Their second son, Zac, born in 1991, was a composite of Brenda and Myles. Zac had Brenda's adventurous spirit—mother and son would later get their motorcycle licenses together, and they would make plans to go skydiving—but he had his father's drive. Zac would struggle in school, just like Myles had, but it was never because the father or the son couldn't do the work. It was because they couldn't feign interest in something that didn't truly interest them. But when something did engage them—math and finance, health and fitness, hunting and football—the father and the son maintained a laser-like focus, and a perfectionism to get things right.

Myles and Brenda had only one son so far when Myles took the coaching job at Simpson College in Indianola, a town just twenty-six miles east of Winterset that was known for monthly motorcycle nights on the town square. Soon after Myles accepted the job came Zac, and a year later, in 1992, their third boy, Levi. All three would play football, but it was the first two sons, Myles II and Zac, who truly adored the sport. On Saturday afternoons in the fall, they'd sneak up to the overhead track at Simpson College's nearly century-old gym and listen to their dad's halftime pep talks. Those talks were legendary for their intensity. After a bad half, Myles would scream things like that the other team was the foxes and "our team" was the rabbits, running away with our tails between our legs. "We're going to let the fox eat us!" he once screamed. "Fucking pussies!" He wasn't afraid to let his players think he was a little unhinged. But what most impressed observers was how he could transition from screaming to teaching. "Okeydokey," he'd say matter-of-factly, marking the end of his expletive-filled rant. "This is what we gotta do." Then, he'd turn to the chalkboard and start diagramming tweaks to their defense.

Daddy Myles valued toughness above all else. It wasn't so much that Zac heard his father preach that mentality and decided to make it his own, though that was certainly part of it. It was more that Zac was born that way. His older brother, Myles II, was taller, faster, talented enough to earn a Division II football scholarship and a spot in his high school's sports hall of fame. Zac was shorter, slower, not as solid. But he was the toughest dude on the field. "Whether it was a guard or a center pulling or a running back coming at him," said Myles II, "Zac was always out there to do some serious damage." Years later, whenever Myles Sr. and II spoke to me about Zac's mindset on the football field, I could hear the awe in their voices.

"Zac, he was always smearing people," said Myles II. "He was just reckless. All the kids in his grade feared him. Not just in football. If you fucked with Zac, he was going to knock you in your mouth. He was jacked, too. We worked out together in the mornings. Me and Zac used to be the type of guys who wanted to knock people out."

"I got the fuck beat out of me in college," Myles Sr. said. "But Zac, man. Wooooo-ooooo. He was a thumper. He loved it."

Of course, that never seemed a big deal at the time. Zac's father had a half dozen or more concussions during his football career; he never seemed worse for the wear. The same held for Zac's older brother. Concussions were just part of the price you paid in this sport that, with the right mentality, could turn you into a man.

Daddy Myles was able to get Zac into youth football a year early, when Zac was in third grade instead of fourth, because he was the coach of the newly formed team. In sixth grade, Zac's team was in the playoffs of the regional youth football league. On one play, Zac, playing linebacker, blitzed the quarterback and sacked him. But he hit the quarterback helmet to helmet. The referee threw a flag, giving Zac a personal foul and the other team a first down on the one-yard line. The other team scored and won the game. Zac cried the entire drive home. That was the only game Daddy Myles and Zac's team lost in two years. The next year, their team won the youth league's Super Bowl.

"Zac and I, when we played, we were hit or sit," his older brother said. "We loved contact more than the other kids."

"Of all the boys, he was the one who wouldn't show pain, who'd be fearless, who'd be calm under pressure," Zac's dad said. "He'd throw his head into anything." He paused thoughtfully. "He was the kind of guy I like on defense."

"I first started having constant headaches while playing youth football and played through it in fear of telling someone, and feeling like a pussy," Zac wrote when he was wrestling with the impact of past concussions. "I started playing youth football a year early in 3rd grade because my older brother was on the team and my dad was the coach. I started off playing the two positions that I played throughout my career, linebacker and full back . . .

"I had gained the reputation from my coaches and classmates about being a tough nosed kid and a hard hitter so I took this social identity with pride and never wanted to tell anyone about the headaches I got from practices and games. In 6th grade, I really

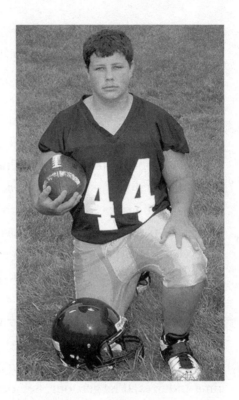

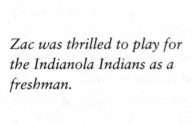

Zac was thrilled to play for the Indianola Indians as a freshman.

became a road grater as a fullback and running back. I was short and chubby, but I would try to run over the linebacker's every time I got the ball. I'm sure my parents still have the game tapes to prove it.

"On one of our last practices that season, I remember going against Dmitry Renneger in a tackling drill. Me and Dmitry always got paired together because we were considered the biggest kids and the most aggressive, but Dmitry was about a foot taller then me so to be able to hold my own I had to use my head as a weapon . . . At the start of the whistle that practice I clashed head on with Big D at full speed. I remember this because it was one of the worst headaches ever and I remember secretly crying for the rest of practice and later at home. I don't know if it was a concussion, but once again it could be questionable now that I look back. [In a] week or so the football season was over and I would say that's when my life started to change. I started getting terrible migraines and neck pain at school and at home. Anything I did would give me a terrible headache and I felt like no one would ever believe me. I remember being teased and feeling like a pussy to my brothers and dad. Finally, I cried to my mom and she started to believe me."

"In the end one of the doctors told my mom it was probably my hormones triggering the migraines and tension headaches."

Myles Sr. read this typewritten autobiography once, after Zac's death, as well as his handwritten journals. He doesn't dwell on them. He hasn't gone to a therapist to work through his grief. He has his own form of therapy: He grabs a few beers and calls for the two dogs. He stalks the family's woods behind their house, shotgun in hand, and when he sees an animal that doesn't belong there, he aims and fires. If he gets one, he notches it on the annual kill list he keeps taped to the family's refrigerator. That's his therapy.

But drowning himself in hunting or alcohol or other diversions is not to say he ignores the sadness of losing a son. He does not talk about it much, but friends noticed that he became deeply, profoundly sad after Zac's death. Nor does he ignore his own role, and the role of the sport he's loved his entire life, in his son's demise.

"I would like football go back to where it was innocent, in the sixties and seventies for me," Myles said. "You knew people got hurt, but you didn't know the lasting effects."

But you can't go back to that more innocent time. Or, perhaps more accurately, that less educated time. Now, we know—and when we know, we cannot ignore. Instead, the father lives with the consequences.

"This all started in youth football," Myles Sr. said. "I wish we had known back then. That's the thing that haunts me. That's the part that really tears me up. We started him in third grade. I think it started way younger than when he was in high school. I know it did. And I don't like to think about it, so I try not to think about it. It'll drive you insane. Because you're supposed to protect them, and you didn't . . . If I'd known, I wouldn't have let him play. Period. There's a toughness thing that would have been lost, a team thing—physical toughness—if he hadn't played football. But that stuff goes out the window because it ruins your body."

He sighed. He closed his eyes. Opened them.

"We didn't know," he said. "We didn't know."

His voice trailed off.

FOUR

The Hammer

THE FINAL DAY of the Iowa State Fair, two Sundays before Labor Day, marks the end of summer in the state. Over the course of eleven days in August 2006, more than a million people walked down the Grand Concourse on the industrial east side of Des Moines; munched on corn dogs and fried Oreos and pork-chops-on-a-stick; browsed the thousands of stalls of farm animals; and headed to the Grandstand for nighttime entertainment. That year's fair featured big country music acts—Brad Paisley, Trace Adkins, Big & Rich—as well as James Taylor. Taylor played on the second night and sang his hit song "Fire and Rain," as the sun set. About a friend who committed suicide, it is perhaps one of the saddest songs ever written.

Moments like that are rare at the Iowa State Fair, a place of fun and frivolity. That August, there were tractor pulls and a stock-car race, and a champion big boar named Waldo that weighed more than a thousand pounds. What made the 2006 fair different than any Iowa State Fair since Myles Easter Sr. had been born in 1961 was that Norma "Duffy" Lyon had retired. For forty-five years, she had sculpted the famed butter cow that stood regally behind glass, as well as other tableaus of Americana: Elvis Presley, *American Gothic*—the painting by Iowa artist Grant Wood—and

John Wayne. During the summer of 2006, Iowans were abuzz at what Lyon's successor, her longtime apprentice Sarah Pratt, would sculpt alongside the butter cow. She chose Superman, since the recently released *Superman Returns* film starred Iowa native Brandon Routh.

The end of summer 2006 marked the beginning of a new chapter for Zac Easter. He would soon be a high school freshman, and by the time the state fair shut its gates on August 20, Zac had already been on the gridiron for the past couple of weeks as a promising new member of the Indianola Indians football team. His older brother, Myles II, was the big, tough senior, a varsity captain who would soon accept a football scholarship at Minnesota State University, Mankato, one of the top Division II programs in the country and where the Minnesota Vikings held their preseason training camp.

When Zac was sized for his helmet that August, the Easter mentality was already accepted as something ingrained in him because it had been ingrained in the team for years through Myles II and their father, the team's defensive coordinator.

Eric Kluver, the head coach, had been hired a few years before, and one of his earliest moves had been to reach out to Myles Easter Sr. He'd felt Myles's toughness would be a perfect addition to his staff. Indianola was a small school compared with many of its conference rivals in the Des Moines suburbs. The bigger schools had twice the students, and more money for facilities and coaches. After a disastrous first season when he opened up the passing attack and played a more skillful, speed-based spread offense, Kluver decided the only way Indianola could compete against larger, stronger, faster schools was by playing in the trenches: by slowing the game down, by out-toughing opponents. As other teams used newfangled pass-happy offenses, Kluver and Myles Sr. turned back the clock to how football was played when they were growing up.

One of Myles Easter's first changes was to punt-return coverage. He was a great tactician on special teams, mostly because special teams can bring the most aggressive and reckless collisions in football. Punts and kickoffs are the most chaotic moments on the field, eleven people sprinting headlong into eleven other people, all primed to lay waste to their opponents. (As the concussion crisis deepened, the NFL revised rules to make those plays less prone to violent collisions.) Myles Easter had blockers form a wall on punt returns, similar to mass-formation plays that created so much controversy in football's early days. By the time Myles was coaching his sons, other teams weren't using walls on punt returns, so that bruising strategy afforded his team a competitive advantage. Indianola's blockers would hit an onrushing defender as hard as they could, then let him run free as the ball carrier dashed past. "You set up a wall, and it's like knocking people off a tee," Myles II said. "If they didn't have their head on a swivel, they were getting fucked up." Sometimes opposing players would be "decleated"— hit so hard their spikes flew off their feet. One of the most memorable plays of Zac's high school career came on a punt return, when he knocked down three people in a row: the Easter mentality distilled into a single ten-second burst.

For a school that had never been known for smashmouth football, this change in philosophy was thrilling. "People would come out in our community just to watch our punt returns," Kluver said. "We would absolutely lay people out. Now, you get flagged for hits like that." What the Indians lacked in size they made up for in heart. They went to an I-formation offense, an old-school style with the quarterback, fullback, and running back bunched together perpendicular to the line of scrimmage. "We needed to shorten the game and control the football and give ourselves a chance to win at the end," Kluver said. "It was a lot of three yards and a cloud of dust."

By the time Zac was a freshman, his older brother's exploits were already legendary. Like any football legend—whether in hulking NFL coliseums or on patches of turf carved into cornfields— Myles II's greatness wasn't fully conveyed by his player profile. To be sure, that profile was impressive. He was a physical, hard-hitting safety who was speedy enough to cover receivers downfield. Once, Myles sprinted from the safety position, smashed the running back in the backfield, popped the ball out, then ran it in for a touchdown. "We were all looking at each other on the sidelines: 'Did he really just do that?'" Kluver recalled. Another time, against suburban powerhouse Ankeny, the opposing running back came out of the backfield on a bubble pass route. The quarterback's throw led him and left him exposed to Myles. Myles hit him so hard, the running back dropped the ball as his cleats popped off his feet. Myles recorded seventy tackles his junior season and eighty-two his senior year, which also included a team-leading five interceptions and one defensive touchdown. Those exploits unanimously nabbed him a spot on the all-conference first team.

But legends aren't made of numbers. Legends are made of bigger-than-life stories. And Myles II had a story of toughness that stood up to generations of Easter men's exploits. He always fought through injuries, but one was particularly gruesome. During a game his junior year, Myles leaned forward to tackle someone, and the runner's knee connected with his bicep. The injury hurt, but he played through it. After the game, his bicep tightened. He couldn't extend his arm. A blood clot, rock hard and the size of a golf ball, had lodged in his bicep. But there was another game the next Friday, so Myles was outfitted with a soft cast and a brace that tugged at his arm to straighten it out. He wore it in class, in practices, in bed. "It sucked, painful as shit," Myles said. "But I felt I could still cover people, still tackle people, so I could still play, even though most people wouldn't have played with just one arm." His right arm was immobilized in a ninety-degree position, so his dad put him on the side of the field where he could tackle with his left arm instead.

During his senior year came another wild injury: An opposing wide receiver ran a crossing route, and Myles went over to smoke him. But the opposing receiver ducked, and Myles flipped over him, his heels hitting the back of his head. He broke the L4 and L5 vertebrae in his lower back. He played the rest of the season with fractured vertebrae. "That's what you do because it's football," he said. "We're a tough family. I could play through it. It wasn't like I had a broken leg and couldn't move."

By the time Zac was a freshman, he'd internalized those lessons his father and brother had taught about how a man was supposed to act.

"Starting freshman football I felt like I had something to prove because my dad was a hard ass football coach and my older brother was a football stud," Zac wrote. "I look back now and can say I always felt [inadequate] as a football player compared to my brother and my father as well and that was a reason I always tried to be tough and play through the pain. There was also the 'Easter Mentality' stereo type that I had to live up to. This 'Easter Mentality' is the name that all the other coaches and kids in sports called us because the Easter family was such a tough nosed football family and the reputation was that football was our lives and we would play through any pain. My dad was an intimidating hard ass football coach and the Easter mentality meant that we were supposed to always be tough as nails, show no weakness, and never get taken out of game for being hurt.

"My freshman year of football I played linebacker and fullback as usual. Once again I literally used my head as a battering ram on every play and even though I was one of the shortest kids on the team, I could kick anyone's ass and run over someone twice my size. My freshman year I also played was plagued by not only constant headaches, but shoulder and neck injuries. Since I lead with my head on every play, I obviously had neck problems which lead to me having tons of stingers and shoulder problems. Coach Tucker would always tell me to quit hitting the hole with my head down, but I never listened because I loved being able to bring it. There were a few games and practices when my stingers got so bad that I could not feel my left arm for a day or two after a game. I also remember one game my freshman year when I had to of had a concussion against Ankeny. I don't remember much of the game, but I remember Joe Hogan telling me about how I couldn't even walk straight during the game and how I couldn't even line up in a three-point stance correctly. We laughed about it when we were watching game tape, but now I look back and wish I could of stopped myself right there."

Even then, before concussions were such a big topic, Indianola coaches taught safety through proper tackling. "See what you hit!" they repeated. "Eyes up!" they drilled. "Run and wrap!" they shouted. Zac heard it all. And he ignored it. "Zac definitely, at times, he'd lower his head—I remember that vividly, not doing exactly what he was coached to do," Kluver recalled. But to Zac, the benefits of using his head as the tip of his body's missile

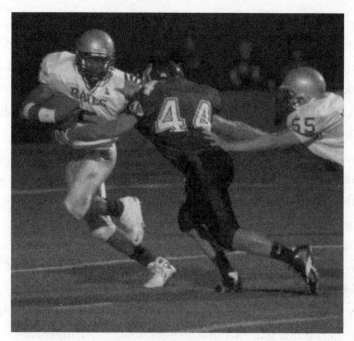

*By his senior year, Zac was a varsity captain,
just like his older brother.*

outweighed any nagging headaches. It was how he made up for his relatively small body. And a way to become a real man.

"Usually, when you have these reckless, crazy athletes, they don't really care," said the school's trainer, Sue Wilson. "They're just stupid and crazy. That was not Zac. He was very passionate about football. He worked hard. Zac always had control of his body. That's different than reckless. Zac was very calculated and controlled. He knew exactly when to use force. He just did it at any cost."

Messages from elders were mixed. Coaches criticized his techniques. They made him wear a cowboy collar, a foam roll around his neck, to force him to hit with his head up. Nick Haworth, one of Zac's best friends, remembers him hearing coaches' criticism:

"That's reckless," coaches would say. "Don't do that." (Later, Haworth would recognize that while coaches admonished Zac, they didn't impose consequences. "Coaches, all they can do is coach," he later told me. "They can't be out there on the field with you.") And even as coaches preached safety, they praised his biggest hits. So did teammates. In the Saturday-morning training room after Friday-night games, teammates would get ice baths while they flipped through the sports pages to hunt for photographs or stories from their game. When they relived their biggest hits, they were often talking about Zac.

"I still take self pride for never pulling myself out of game," Zac wrote. "I was tougher than nails. Everyone on the team looked up to me as the leader and being tough. I played every game with a constant headache, and I remember one game against Knoxville where I got dinged so hard that after the game I hid in the locker room during the varsity game and cried because my head hurt so bad."

Kluver had a tradition: to give a T-shirt emblazoned with the words BIG HAMMER to the player who doled out the game's most punishing hit. BIG HAMMER T-shirts were coveted, a physical talisman of warrior-like courage. In high school, Zac won two. Later, once the fear of traumatic brain injuries cast a cloud over football—and once the hits that won BIG HAMMER T-shirts started getting flagged as illegal—Kluver stopped handing them out. He felt remorse: "Maybe that shouldn't have been a reward," he lamented. But for years afterward, BIG HAMMER shirts still appeared in the halls of Indianola High School, passed down from older brothers to younger brothers. Players would nudge Kluver about it: "How come we don't get those shirts?" Implicit in their question was that their test of manhood was weaker than that of their predecessors.

Zac's hard-hitting mentality had gained him notice since before he could walk: He loved putting his body in danger's way. He was reckless on jet skis. He was nutty when he climbed trees. He was fearless on the four-wheeler, confident that, no matter how fast he pushed it, he would always be in control—and would never get hurt. "That's what you want on a football team," his father said. Once, Zac and his father were riding the four-wheeler together at night when they misjudged a hill near a creek bed. "Get off!" Myles Sr. shouted. Zac pushed himself off the back of the four-wheeler. His dad landed on his head with the all-terrain vehicle on top of him. His head was bleeding. "Zac rolled it off me and said, 'You all right?'" his father recalled. He was fine, though the scar was permanent. "That is *not* funny," Brenda told them. The boys laughed anyway. She was always trying to protect her boys from danger, but a mother of three Easter boys quickly came to realize it was a fruitless fight.

As Zac's football collisions came against players exponentially bigger, stronger, and faster than those he'd mauled in his youth, Zac's ability to hide the effects of his injuries waned. At one point, a friend told the trainer Zac's stingers—a nerve injury that often occurs during tackling, when the shoulder gets forced one way and the head and neck the other way—had gotten so bad he couldn't feel his left arm. Wilson made him sit out a few games.

"Once I realized telling them the truth would make me half to sit out," Zac wrote, "I stopped telling them and often lied about ever injury."

His junior year, Zac tore a quad and missed a few games. Once he was back, he pledged to hit harder than ever. Teammates teased him about being a dirty player because on every play, Zac hit as hard as he could, even if he didn't have to. By the time Zac was a senior in late summer 2009, he was a varsity captain like his older brother had been. "He was the next Easter in line," Kluver said. "He wanted to live up to that Easter name."

During Zac's junior year, Sue Wilson, the trainer, spotted something weird. During one game, she noticed Zac's left arm hung limply to one side. His head was tilted to the same side. Zac had been on her radar for years as a high-risk player. From the first time she saw him play, she noticed that he led with his head. When she told him he needed to tackle with his head up, his answer was scary: "I don't know how. I don't know how to be powerful with my head up." So when she saw him running lopsidedly during that game his junior year, she approached him. "Sue, it hurts bad," Zac told her. She asked why his head was tilted. "It's not," he said. It was. He couldn't tell; he thought his head was perfectly vertical. She walked to the coach and said: "He's done." He sat out the rest of that game. Doctors later noted his brachial plexus, a network of nerves that stretches from the neck down to the top rib and into the armpit, was pulling away from the spinal column.

By the summer of 2009, most of high school had flown by. Zac was a popular jock, but he was never a bully, never a jerk. Like Odie from *Garfield and Friends*, Zac was friends with everybody. He was excited for his final season. The week before practices started, Zac and his father caravanned with others three hours southeast to Kirksville, Missouri, for a padded, full-contact football camp at Truman State University. Zac was going against players from other states, so he could impress college coaches while making a statement to teammates that this season would be *his* time. He teed off on opponents at every opportunity. At one point, Zac was trying to lay a big hit on a ball carrier. He lowered his head, and . . . BAM! Helmet to helmet. The noise was so loud that players winced—"OH!"—and other campers turned their heads to see who got crunched. "Zac came off to the side, and he looked dizzy," his friend Haworth recalled. "He was really quiet. He didn't want to say anything. He knew he'd get taken out. Zac never wanted to appear weak, and if you had to sit out, he thought it made you look pretty weak, like you couldn't hack it."

"I remember getting my concussion the second day of camp during the very first tackling drill of the morning," Zac wrote. "We were doing an outside linebacker rip and tackle drill. I was even holding a bag, but I still lead with my head to smoke this ball carrier who was from a different team. I put him on his ass, but could barely stand up right after. The headache was so intense I could barely talk to anyone. As usual, I sucked it up and practiced the whole time and made sure I never let up to show any weakness on ever play. I was so mentally engrained on being the toughest baddest that I almost started to take pleasure in having a pounding headache and still bringing it on ever play . . . By the last scrimmage that day, I could barely walk or call the plays, and once again it was my best friends who told the coaches."

Zac was held out of contact drills the rest of camp. But when the high school team held its first practice a week later, there Zac was, ready to play football. He was eighteen years old and invincible. As Haworth would say later, "They wanted us to be tough guys, hard-ass and tough. And it's hard to be tough when you're standing on the sidelines." For a few days, Zac complained to his older brother that his head hurt. At home after school, he lay down and put a towel over his face. "Then, he popped out of it and seemed normal," Myles II recalled. "His neck was fucked up. But he just played the whole year like that."

"When I got home [from the preseason camp] I saw a doctor and lied about all my concussion symptoms," Zac wrote. "I

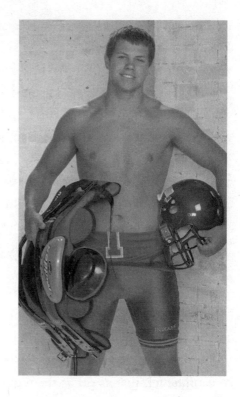

Zac was conscious of his body image and obsessed with working out.

continued practice before the season with terrible headaches and never said a word to anyone."

The second concussion of Zac's senior year came on the night of the fourth game, in mid-September. Knowing Zac's history and his mindset, Sue Wilson was nervous. But his primary care physician had cleared him to play, and he certainly wanted to play. During the game, Wilson kept a close eye on him. On one play, Zac smashed against an opponent, a loud helmet-to-helmet hit. Wilson heard it from the other end of the field and walked toward him. His head was down. He staggered, then fell. "Sue, Zac needs you," a teammate said. Zac jogged to the sidelines, pretending everything was all right. "Look at me," Wilson instructed. He tried to zero in on her, but he couldn't. "Your eyes are all over the place," she told him. "Where are you?" Zac just shook his head. "Are you going to throw up?" He shook his head again. "You're done," she said.

A coach came over to Wilson, seemingly brushing off the situation: "He just got his bell rung, right?" At the end of the quarter, she went back to Zac and stared in his eyes. They were still darting about, something called saccades, rapid and simultaneous movements of both eyes, as opposed to the smooth movements eyes normally make together. It was a muscle-control issue in the brain, convincing evidence Zac was concussed.

"I want to go back in," Zac told her.

"It's not an option."

"This is why I don't tell you anything."

"Your coaches know you're done," Wilson told Zac, taking his helmet. "Don't try to get back on the field."

When he came into the trainer's office the next morning, he told Wilson he felt just as off as the night before. The symptoms hadn't cleared up. "I just feel weird," he said. Wilson told him to rest, and that he wouldn't play in the next game.

At this point, Zac certainly knew stories of ex-football players struggling with bad knees or bum shoulders. But you could live with that, the price of becoming a man. He had never heard of the disease that would soon change the way Americans thought about football. During Zac's freshman year, in January 2007, Alan Schwarz of the *New York Times* had published the first piece in mainstream American media that indicated a connection between playing football and sustaining brain damage. The article was about Andre Waters, a hard-hitting NFL safety for twelve seasons who committed suicide a decade after retiring. But suicide could come from any number of causes; Zac's own father reasoned that a rash of high-profile suicides of NFL players in the late 2000s was probably because retired players struggled with living life out of the spotlight. In September of Zac's senior year, *GQ* magazine published a piece by Jeanne Marie Laskas that profiled a young Pittsburgh neuropathologist named Bennet Omalu. That story would eventually be adapted for the Will Smith movie *Concussion*, about a Nigerian immigrant who researched connections between football and brain injuries and battled the mighty NFL.

But by Zac's senior year, the concern about connections between concussions in football and debilitating brain damage had yet to reach a fever pitch. And when he graduated from high school and ended his football career, Zac Easter had never once heard of the neurodegenerative disease that was taking root in his brain.

BY THE TIME Cyndy Feasel first heard of CTE, it was too late. Far too late.

Her name was Cyndy Davy when she met Grant Feasel at Abilene Christian University in the near-desert of West Texas. He was a towering six-foot-seven, strong-jawed California kid whose boyish good looks brought to mind John F. Kennedy Jr., the former president's son. He hoped to become a dentist, but the allure of football diverted him from that, even after being accepted at Texas Southwestern Medical School. He'd played since age eight. The sport got him a full ride to a university he otherwise couldn't afford, and it also offered him a chance at whatever measure of fame and fortune could be earned by a center, whose profession is to snap the ball between his legs, then push, claw, and shove at opponents trying to tackle the man with the ball.

Grant and Cyndy married in 1983 while they were both still in college. "It was everything I'd dreamed of, just an instant connection of love and respect," Cyndy said. They were both excited when the Baltimore Colts chose Grant as the 161st selection in the 1983 NFL draft. This was the moment he could have left football behind and pursued his longtime dream of a career in dentistry, but the sport's glory had a magnetic pull. "He kept going back to the game," Cyndy told me. "There's a thrill to it. It's the ultimate guys' club."

And let's be honest: Cyndy was thrilled, too. Like any self-respecting Texan, the brown-eyed blonde had grown up around football. After games, she'd ask Grant about what had really happened in the trenches, and he was elated to relive his anonymous offensive line battles. Being a center and long snapper is not glamorous. It's a position that meant he banged heads with opponents on virtually every play as a rookie with the Colts, then with the Minnesota Vikings, and, finally, with the Seattle Seahawks. During his near-decade in the NFL, Feasel would have snapped the ball between his legs and then risen to bash helmets somewhere on the order of ten thousand times in games, plus who knows how many times in practices. But he and Cyndy were living an idyllic all-American life: the football player, his beautiful wife, and their growing family.

Cyndy first noticed a disconnect when she was pregnant and Grant hurt his leg in a game. "I wouldn't have gotten injured if I wasn't worried about you having a baby," he told her. Strange: The comment came across as angry, and very un-Grant. Then came the drinking and pain pills. Everywhere he went, he kept a handful of Advil in his pocket. The Percocet prescribed by team doctors helped with the constant pain and helped him sleep. Over time, his heavy drinking progressed into full-blown alcoholism. He retired from the Seahawks in 1993 and got a sales job with a company that made digital X-ray and mammography equipment. He mostly stayed holed up in his home office in Fort Worth answering e-mails, returning sales calls, and drinking Absolut Vodka from forty-four-ounce Styrofoam Route 44 cups he'd saved from Sonic Drive-In.

It was as if Grant was slowly disappearing from their marriage. Cyndy fought the loss. When she came across booze, she'd pour the 1.75-liter bottles down the drain. Grant got a minifridge for his closet, and Cyndy raided that. too. So Grant put his fridge under lock and key. His body deteriorated. His hands shook, so he'd keep them in his pockets, thinking nobody would notice. A psychiatrist prescribed Xanax for anxiety; Grant ground the pills up, mixed them in vodka and finished the hundred-pill prescription in a week.

He became gaunt, his eyes sunken. A doctor said he needed to get to a rehab facility, and soon. He became paranoid, and occasionally physically abusive as well. As Cyndy recalls the situation, the abuse began when he found her snooping in his closet. He feared she was going after his alcohol, so he shoved her to the ground. It only got worse when Grant learned of an affair that Cyndy, distraught in the marriage, had with another man. "I was devastated—my husband had chosen alcohol over our family our entire marriage," Cyndy said. "Grant would say, 'You're a fucking whore.' He'd say this to our kids' faces. He'd say, 'You've cheated on me your whole life. You cheated on me before we got married.' And all I ever did was love him!"

By 2010, seventeen years after his career ended, their marriage had fully come apart. Cyndy was scared of her husband: his anger, his drunk driving, his mental deterioration. At times, though, he was lucid. When he needed a drink, he'd be angry or feisty; moments of lucidity, and of kindness, came when he was hammered. One night, when he was drunk and calm, Cyndy asked if he was going back to rehab. "No, I'm done with it," Grant told her. "I think I have what Mike had." He meant Mike Webster, the Pittsburgh Steelers Hall of Fame center whom Grant idolized. Webster had died in 2002 after a long and terrifying descent—from NFL legend to a bankrupt, homeless, and depressed shell of himself, and able to sleep only after shocking himself with a Taser. Webster's deteriorated brain became the basis of Omalu's research into brain damage among former NFL players.

"Did you have a lot of concussions?" she asked him.

"Hundreds."

Her mind swirled. She walked to the nightstand and scribbled his words on a notepad. Maybe something more was going on here than the anger and confusion of an old ballplayer who missed his football days.

The end of their marriage came in the wee hours one day at 3:00 a.m. They had long ago devolved to having separate bedrooms, and Grant burst into Cyndy's room, knife in hand. "I just called the police," he said. Her first thought was he'd done something awful—hurt someone, killed someone—but then she realized the drama was all in his mind. "I told the police you're trying to kill me," Grant said. She escaped into a bathroom, locked the door, and called the police. The next day, Cyndy moved into a friend's townhouse.

Even after the divorce, Cyndy didn't sever all ties. After learning Grant was in the hospital for cirrhosis of the liver, she'd leave the elementary school where she worked as an art teacher to visit him over her lunch hour. One of the final times she saw him was in a hospital room. He was fiddling with an old flip phone, unable to get it to work. It was a devastating portrait of a broken man, fired from his job, prone in a hospital bed, frustrated like a toddler who couldn't get his cell phone to work. She crawled in next to him. "I've loved you all these years," she told him. "It just makes me sad how it all ended. I'm sorry, sorry for everything." And Grant said, "I'm sorry for everything, too." Not long after, he moved into hospice. He died July 15, 2012, at age fifty-two. The official cause was cirrhosis of the liver.

Grant's family donated his brain to the Concussion Legacy Foundation, and doctors sliced it up to determine if something more than a fondness for alcohol was behind Grant's demise. When Cyndy read the official autopsy report, she was floored. He had chronic traumatic encephalopathy, or CTE, the degenerative brain disease found in the brains of other former NFL players who'd died relatively young, many from suicide. His brain was one of 111 brains of deceased former NFL players in the study that Dr. Ann McKee, director of the Boston University CTE Center, would later publish in the *Journal of the American Medical Association*. Of those brains, 110 showed signs of CTE, including Grant's. His brain had so deteriorated that he was already considered Stage 3 out of a possible four stages. A doctor told Cyndy that Grant would have been virtually "mindless" within a year.

In the simplest of terms, the brain disease that's upended the sport of football can be thought of as brain scarring, either from big, explosive hits that result in concussions, or from repetitive sub-concussive hits that players like linemen—like Mike Webster, like Grant Feasel—receive on every single play. The brain is not fixed in the head. It's an incredibly complicated piece of human hardware, a spongy mass of tissue that's six inches long in an adult and weighs three pounds. It's swimming in cerebrospinal fluid inside the skull. Some areas of the brain can be susceptible to tearing when a force rattles and bangs it against the skull walls. The wrinkles you see in images of a human brain are either ridge-like folds, which are known as gyri, or the crevices between those folds, known as sulci. While CTE has similar outward-facing characteristics as Alzheimer's disease, the proteins that cause Alzheimer's accumulate all over the folds and crevices of the brain. In CTE, which is caused by brain cells essentially tearing, bad proteins accumulate deep in those crevices in the brain's gray matter.

All human brains have something called tau proteins that stabilize connections in the brain. They give structural integrity to pathways that connect neurons, which receive signals from the brain and spinal cord to direct the actions of the human body to axons, the long, slender nerve fibers that transmit the neurons' instructions throughout the body.

Think of the brain as a functioning subway system whose job is to transport electrical impulses to operate the body. The cell bodies of each neuron are like a subway hub—say, Grand Central Station. The axon, or nerve fiber, is like a subway tunnel, where electrical impulses are transported away from the neuron. Proteins called kinesin and dynein are like subway cars that transport other proteins from the neuron; like two separate tracks of a subway heading in opposite ways, kinesin goes in one direction while dynein goes in the opposite direction. Inside axon-tunnels are subway tracks. The tracks consist of two things: microtubules, like beams of a railroad track, and tau proteins, the planks holding the track together and stabilizing the beams. Electrical impulses are transported up and down these tracks to run the human body. When the brain is exposed to tearing, more tau proteins are released. And when there's a massive buildup of tau proteins over time— when the planks that hold together the railway begin to clump together and clog things up—the ability to transmit electrical impulses is diminished. CTE is like a massive traffic backup on the brain-subway.

"Researching a human brain is not a bloody, messy experience," said Dr. Kevin Bieniek, a neuropathologist at UT Health San Antonio who studies CTE. "It's a very neat organ, with all these different boundaries and markings in its structure. When you take a step back and think about this piece of tissue I'm looking at was responsible for every facet of a person's life, consciousness and being, it's pretty deep stuff."

Cyndy Feasel didn't understand the science of her husband's clogged brain cells. But it was easy to understand the overall picture: Repeated blows to the head had scarred his brain beyond repair.

For Cyndy, the news about Grant's autopsy was devastating. But at least it was an explanation for the dramatic changes in his personality. In that sense, it was somewhat relieving. Cyndy was grateful to finally put a name to the disease that destroyed her husband, and hopeful the NFL would fight the disease. "There had been no answers," Cyndy said. "And then the minute I saw the autopsy report, I realized it coincided with every story in my journals, every story that said, 'Where did Grant go? Where is the man I married?'"

Cyndy dove into an Internet dark hole. She learned CTE was brought into the public consciousness by Omalu, who'd discovered a buildup of tau proteins in the brain of Mike Webster, Grant's football idol. She read Jeanne Marie Laskas's story in *GQ*, and she learned Omalu had studied brains of other former NFL players with signs of CTE. Omalu's second brain was that of former Steelers guard Terry Long, who died at age forty-five after drinking antifreeze; it looked like a ninety-year-old's brain torn apart by

Alzheimer's. The third brain was that of Andre Waters, who shot himself in the head at age forty-four. The fourth brain was that of Justin Strzelcyzyk, another former Steelers lineman who at age thirty-six, after ranting and raving at a gas station near Buffalo, led a forty-mile chase by police before swerving into oncoming traffic and smashing into a tanker truck. The brains kept coming, and the circumstances were eerily similar: Former NFL players whose lives and sanity quickly deteriorated after their careers ended. Then, they died, often young and dramatically.

Omalu's original paper, published in 2005 in *Neurosurgery* with five coauthors and titled "Chronic Traumatic Encephalopathy in a National Football League Player," laid out the science that the kind of repetitive blows to the head that NFL players experience could cause debilitating brain damage.

It would make sense if, on the heels of the article's publication, the NFL had mustered its considerable forces to fight the disease. Except that wasn't the case at all. Cyndy was distraught to learn that instead of fighting the disease, the NFL spent a decade or so *fighting the research* (and the researchers). She read how the league had rejected Omalu's scientific claims from the start. She learned the NFL's concussion crisis was like so many controversies in modern-day America, which meant that discussions about facts and science quickly morphed into discussions about politics and money and power.

And then Cyndy Feasel became enraged.

The image of the old, beaten-down, retired football player is nearly as ingrained in the American consciousness as the image of the heroic, virile young gladiator in a suit of pads and a masked helmet. Since the beginning of the game, football injuries were badges of courage. So you had a bum knee or a bad limp? That meant you were a warrior, and this was proof. But *brain damage?* That was different. *How can the brain be hurt by football when these warriors are so armored up with those protective helmets?* Cyndy wondered.

Well, about those helmets: The first football helmet was likely invented in 1893 by a midshipman at the United States Naval Academy named Joseph Reeves. The lineman was nicknamed "Bull" because on the playing field he was undersized but overpowering. And Bull led with his head. Navy was about to play Army on December 2, 1893, and a school physician warned Reeves, who had a history of head injuries, that his next head shot could cause "instant insanity," even death. The academy superintendent barred Reeves from playing.

But this was the Army-Navy game, which was quickly becoming a highlight of the American sporting calendar. Reeves *had* to play. So he went to a shoemaker and fashioned his own padded moleskin cap. Navy won, and Reeves not only survived the game but excelled later, becoming an admiral in the United States Navy. (That 1893 game, incidentally, nearly led to a duel between a general and an admiral caught up in the hysterics of the rivalry; because of that, the Army-Navy game was canceled for the next five years.)

But the fact that Reeves made it through his final football game without a major brain injury and went on to an illustrious military career is not the point. The point is this: The first indication from a doctor that the contact regularly sustained in football could lead to debilitating brain injuries happened 109 years before Mike Webster's death, and 112 years before the publication of Omalu's paper, and 118 years and five months before Junior Seau's suicide, a paradigm-shifting event that was followed, seventy-four days later, by Grant Feasel's death, his liver ruined and brain shattered.

In fact, the idea that a brain rattling inside the skull could do long-term damage goes back centuries. The author Jeanne Marie Laskas traces research into brain ailments like CTE to "the Father of Medicine," Hippocrates, some four centuries BC. Hippocrates called it *commotio cerebri*, or ailments resulting from "commotion of the brain." The first to use to term *cerebral concussion* was the tenth-century Persian physician Abu Bakr Muhammad ibn Zakariya Razi; he was referring to a brain injury more subtle than the type that could immediately kill you, instead one that made you dizzy or unconscious but that you'd recover from. In sixteenth-century Italy, a physician named Jacopo Berengario da Capri correctly hypothesized concussions were caused by the brain's soft tissue smacking against the skull's hard walls. In the early 1900s, two New York neuropsychiatrists named Michael Osnato and Vincent Giliberti found degenerative mental illnesses in patients who'd sustained concussions. This was the first scientific theory that suggested concussions were an "actual cerebral injury," as the two neuropsychiatrists wrote in a 1927 issue of the *Journal of the American Medical Association*: "It is no longer possible to say that 'concussion is an essentially transient state which does not comprise any evidence of structural cerebral injury.'"

The next year, in 1928, Harrison Martland, the medical examiner in Essex County, New Jersey, coined the term *punch drunk* to describe symptoms associated with repeated head trauma. He'd been studying boxers who late in their careers started acting strangely—or, as fans derided them, "cuckoo," "goofy" or "slug nutty." He wrote of one fight that was stopped because the referee thought a fighter was drunk. The article presumed this condition was mostly limited to boxers: "Punch drunk most often affects fighters of the slugging type, who are usually poor boxers and who take considerable head punishment, seeking only to land a knock-out blow. It is also common in second rate fighters used for training purposes, who may be knocked down several times a day."

Martland's study posited a direct connection between boxing and brain injuries because nearly 50 percent of the boxers he'd studied came down with these symptoms "if they keep at the game long enough." In retrospect, after the recent spate of stories of CTE-damaged NFL brains, Martland's description of "punch drunk" nearly a century ago is chilling: "In severe cases, there may develop a peculiar tilting of the head, a marked dragging of one or both legs, a staggering, propulsive gait with the facial characteristics of parkinsonian syndrome, or a backward swaying of the body, tremors, vertigo and deafness. Finally, marked mental deterioration may set in, necessitating commitment to an asylum."

While boxing was at that time, in the Roaring Twenties, one of America's most popular sports, football—specifically, collegiate football—was as well. That same year, 1928, John R. Tunis, the famed American sports author and broadcaster, wrote an essay in *Harper's* titled "The Great God Football," attacking football as "almost our national religion." It's stunning that during the intervening decades a deeper connection wasn't made between the risk of head injuries in boxing and the risk of head injuries in football. A more scientific-sounding name for what had been called punch drunk was coined in 1937: *dementia pugilistica*. All the research, however, was limited to boxers. Despite the medical concerns, America loved boxing, so the fights went on. In 1943, however, Martland stated this boxers' disease might also be found in wrestlers, perhaps even in football players.

In retrospect, though, it is remarkable that it took until Bennet Omalu published an article in 2005 for Americans to begin to correlate football and CTE. Football is, of course, a sport we have long worshipped for the exact type of high-impact hits that can contribute to this disease. American sports have long differentiated between "necessary roughness" and "unnecessary roughness." The unnecessary version was the type of violence that was outside the bounds of good taste, and against the rules of the game. But football's violence has always seemed of the necessary variety—not freak accidents but a vital part of why we love the game. This is what makes the current situation football's existential crisis, because the collisions that occur regularly are linked with the development of neurodegenerative brain disease. As Ann McKee, director of the Boston University CTE Center, has stated, "I am wondering if, on some level, if every single football player doesn't have this."

When Cyndy Feasel learned of the NFL's response, a denial that started with three NFL-paid doctors demanding a retraction of Omalu's original article in *Neurosurgery*—they wrote it had "serious flaws" and was a "complete misunderstanding" of science—she was stunned. Instead of the usual cycle of humans grappling over and being perplexed by new scientific research, the response felt like willful ignorance. This response was far more egregious than new NFL commissioner Paul Tagliabue's comments in 1989, marking the first official NFL statement on the danger of concussions. "This is one of those pack journalism issues, frankly," Tagliabue had said. "The problem is a journalist issue."

As CTE research turned into a torrent, it became apparent this was more than a "pack journalism" issue. Yet for years, NFL opposition to Omalu's findings continued, as the organization deemed his research "preposterous" or "purely speculative." In a 2007 interview on HBO's *Real Sports*, a cochair of the NFL's Mild Traumatic Brain Injury committee was asked if repeated concussions suffered in football could result in brain damage, dementia, or depression. He answered no six different times. The NFL promoted dubious science to discount football-related concussion concerns. The efforts to distance football from CTE began to resemble the tobacco industry distancing smoking from cancer.

Cyndy Feasel went through a range of emotions when she learned about the disease found in Grant's brain: first relieved, then enraged, then determined to take action. She felt it was her duty to speak out. But this was David vs. the ultimate Goliath. She wasn't just up against the NFL. She was one lonely female voice against an ingrained culture of football machismo that stemmed from an industry worth billions, a giant that was a vital part of American consumer culture and the American education system, that had been part of our national DNA since not long after the Civil War. It blew her away that despite the research about football and CTE, Americans still swore by the sport. It was as if football fans didn't consider players' humanity. "We're still addicted," she said. "It's ingrained in our life, in our society at all levels." Maybe it comes down to this: When we love something so deeply, we justify any number of reasons why the thing we love isn't so bad.

Cyndy assumed one voice couldn't make a difference. But certainly, there had to be more like hers. So she wrote a book detailing how CTE ruined her family. Not long after it was published, she got a call from another widow of an NFL player with CTE. "There's thousands of us out here," she told Cyndy.

THE FIRST-PERIOD BELL rang at 8:00 a.m. on the second Friday in October 2009, just as Iowa farmers were beginning to harvest that season's record corn crop. Indianola High School is a large, low-slung, sprawling red-brick building that encapsulates the town's place in the world: too small to be considered a suburban power-house, too big to be put in the same quaint and charming bucket as other Iowa small towns. Indianola is far enough from Des Moines to have its own ecosystem but close enough to be considered as being in the big city's orbit.

That morning, Indianola's football players were already in a foul mood. They would be playing Ankeny High School in the evening, one of the biggest high schools in Iowa in a city the United States Census Bureau has identified as the fastest-growing in the Midwest. Ankeny also boasted one of the most successful football programs in the state. Every year Zac had been in high school, his team had been pummeled by that suburban school. But there was reason to think that this time, during Zac's senior year, might be different. Ankeny was 5–1, but Indianola was 4–2, a strong start for this gritty, tough team shaped in the Easter image.

Cheerleaders made signs for the players' lockers and brought them cookies. But the signs and sweets didn't lift the players' dark, belligerent moods. "We were ready to play the game at 8:00 a.m.," Zac's friend, Nick Haworth, recalled. "None of us were in the mood to talk." The reticence wasn't just because Ankeny was good. It was more that . . . Well, listen to Haworth: "We just thought they were kind of rich pricks. When they hand out that scouting report and it says Ankeny, a little hair stands up on the back of your neck . . . It was one of those schools that rubbed us the wrong way. They were big jaw-jackers. We were just from a small town. It was almost like we had chips always stacked against us." Beating Ankeny could be something to relive at reunions for decades. Hell, even if they lost, they wanted the Ankeny football players to feel it in their aching bones afterward.

So of course Zac Easter—senior football player, team captain, the latest heir to the Easter mentality that had developed over seven generations in this slice of middle America—was juiced. It would be his first game in a month, since the concussion that had knocked him out. Zac was still hurting, but he would be fully armored up, a soldier heading into battle. He was wearing that cowboy collar, and now he was outfitted with a special Xenith helmet his father had ordered, which was supposed to reduce the risk of concussion. Zac had passed the concussion protocol before being cleared for the game, but trainer Sue Wilson had no idea that Zac had faked his way through testing. She had no idea he'd been lying to his doctors since summer, when he had that concussion at the camp in Missouri. (It wouldn't be until the next season that the Iowa High School Athletic Association would give schools a consistent and rigorous protocol treatment for athletes who may have suffered a concussion.)

This is what Zac wrote about how his body reacted in the months after that concussion: "I remember feeling extremely dizzy through out the rest of the season and sometimes I would fall over in the locker room taking off my pads . . . Either the first or second game I got another bad concussion during the game. I don't really remember much except I didn't get pulled out of the game until I could barely get up and walk. My buddy Nick told me that at one point I looked at him cross eyed."

Zac's parents took him to doctors. They were concerned, sure, but Zac was tough. He could get over a ding or two to the head. And when doctors cleared him, it never occurred to his parents that Zac had simply lied his way through the appointment.

"The truth was I had severe headaches every day and constantly felt sick or dizzy, but the tough guy in me told them I was still totally fine," he wrote. "I remember leaving some of my classes because I would be feeling sick and sitting there soaking myself in sweat. Around this time is when I started feeling depressed. I felt ashamed that I was hurt and had to sit out. I don't know exactly what I felt, but this is when I think I started to never be the same Zac Easter. After like 2 weeks I finally got to play in the next game against Ankeny. I remember getting another terrible headache during the first practice back and even my friends noticed that week that I wasn't as willing to hit as hard and I would actually shy away from contact."

Zac's older brother was in the stands, ready to cheer on his two younger brothers, Zac and Levi. Myles Easter II had transferred to Grand View University, a small, private liberal arts school in Des Moines, and played football there; he wanted to get more playing time. One good part of being closer to home was he could make all Zac's senior-year games. And so he settled into the stands on the chilly October night, greeted old friends, and waited for his brother's return to the gridiron.

The sun had just set, and the lights shone bright: Friday night lights, what the Easter family lived for. Indianola didn't yet have a proper high school field, so they were playing at Simpson College as usual. Before the game, Kluver rounded the team up in the old Hopper gymnasium, the same century-old gym with the overhead track where Zac and his brothers used to run around as little boys and listen to their father's rousing halftime speeches. Before this game, all the players got silent. You could hear a pin drop. That's how Kluver gets his players to focus. It felt like a meditation, warriors readying for battle, until the players exploded, all shouting and clapping and testosterone, and walked as a team down the steep stairs and toward the gridiron, spikes clicking against concrete in unison.

Zac was fired up. Sue Wilson was not. She planned to keep a close eye on Zac. She had been hired in 2005, the same year Bennet Omalu and five coauthors published their paper about his studies of Mike Webster's brain. One of Wilson's primary focuses was concussions, and from the moment she set foot on the football field as the new lady in town, coaches and parents and players thought she was just bringing new problems. When she arrived, the worry about violent contact sports causing brain damage was barely a murmur. But by 2009, the murmur was increasing. Justin Strzelczyk had committed suicide in 2004, and Andre Waters had committed suicide in 2006. One month before Zac took the field for what would be his final high school football game, Jeanne Marie Laskas published her profile on Omalu in *GQ* magazine. That said, Dave Duerson's suicide would not be for another two years, Junior Seau's not for another three years. The federal class-action lawsuit by former NFL players against the league would not be filed for a couple more years. If concern at the highest levels was real and increasing, that concern had not yet fully reached Indianola High School.

"During the Ankeny game I remember the first play of the game is when I got my bell seriously rung," Zac later wrote. "I don't remember anything form the game except from the game tape and from what friends tell me. I went head to head with the running back at full speed on the first play during a quarter back rollout to try and run him over. I could of ripped through the running back and made a sack, instead I wanted to punish this running back on the first play and get inside his head. Instead he got inside of mine, I never pulled myself out of the game though and Chia [a teammate] told me that during halftime he remembered me trying to take a knee in the locker room and I fell over because I was so

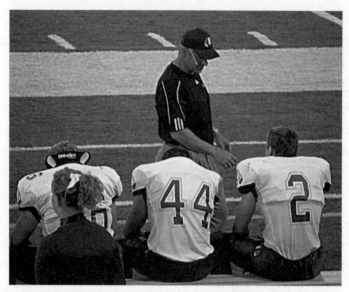

Myles Easter Sr. was the defensive coordinator,
and Zac (No. 44) was a defensive star.

disorientated and I couldn't get back up without a friend helping. Ofcourse I told him I was fine and showed no weakness."

The worst thing immediately after a big hit to the brain is another big hit. And yet, after halftime, there was Zac Easter, walking out of old Hopper gymnasium, his spikes *click-click-click*ing as he made his way to the playing field. His team was losing, but it was a tough, low-scoring game, well within reach, the type of game that favored Indianola. He needed to be out there with his teammates. *For* his teammates.

"It wasn't long during the 3rd quarter when my helmet came off during a play and I guess I hit a guy without a helmet on, head to head," Zac later wrote. "The next play I shit canned a pulling guard and that's about all I remember. From what I was told I could barely get up and wasn't able to walk off the field on my own."

It happened away from the ball, so the collision that ended Zac Easter's football career can't be seen on game tape. "He just smoked this guy who was twice the size of him," his older brother recalled. "He got up and he was wobbling. He had no clue where he was walking. I was like, 'Oh shit, this is not good.'" Two teammates pulled a player off the ground and dragged him toward Wilson. When she saw his jersey number, 44, her heart dropped into her stomach. Zac's feet were barely under him.

"Sue, he's not right," one teammate said.

Zac didn't say a word. He sat on the bench and put his head down. He started crying. He could still speak, he could still stick his tongue out, and he wasn't vomiting. Even though his head was pounding, he didn't seem in need of urgent medical attention.

Years later, I sat in my basement, watching and rewinding game tape from that night. I saw Zac all over the place, often jumping right into pileups on the field. But on that third-quarter drive, I could tell that number 44 was suddenly missing from Indianola's defense. Later in the game, at the bottom of the screen, Zac could be seen on the sidelines, arguing heatedly with someone: Wilson, the trainer. She was clutching his helmet. He wanted to go back in. Kluver came over. Zac had his hands on his hips. He was trying to talk her into letting him go back in.

"No way," she said.

A nearly full moon was rising as the players walked off the field after their 24–9 loss. In the locker room, Zac's blue eyes drifted into a haze. "A thousand-yard stare," Nick Haworth called it. Nobody wanted to talk after a loss, especially to Ankeny. Haworth walked up to his friend. "I could tell Zac wasn't there," he recalled. "It was like a blank stare. I'm like, 'Zac? Dude, what's going on?' And he said, 'Nothing, man, I'm all good.' It was almost like he didn't want to say too much because if he started throwing words together, he may get exposed. I got my shit packed up. We walked out of the locker room together, and I said, 'Hey man, we're going to go see Sue.' 'No, man. We don't need to.' 'You're fucking going with me, and we're going to see Sue.'"

Haworth grabbed his friend's arm and sat him down on the examination table in the trainer's office. "Sue, he's not right," Haworth said.

Years later, Zac wrote about what followed: "It didn't take long before I realized something had changed in me. For the few months the headaches were a daily thing and I always felt sick. I started feeling really depressed and lonely. I had lost football and I felt like I was socially off. I stopped going to any high school events and didn't wrestle that year. Most nights I would sit at home in my basement with the lights off . . . People noticed that I had lost my sense of humor and I would sit in class dead quiet with a blank stair."

He started cheating in class. He cheated on the ACT test.

"I answered some, but my head was killing me. I also started to get super sensitive and felt sensitive to everything. I stopped being the class goof off and started becoming the quiet kid so I wouldn't get anyone's attention. Now that I look back I think it's safe to say that I just felt miserable because I was never the same person I used to be."

A month or two after the third concussion of Zac's senior year, he approached Wilson about being on the wrestling team.

"You're done," she told him. "I'm sorry, but I won't clear you."

"Will other doctors?"

"I hope not."

"I'll never forget the look in Zac's eyes when I told him that," Wilson recalled. "I think his exact words were 'Fuck you.'"

"I really don't even remember much of that year," Zac wrote. "I mainly only remember the events that friends have since told me about, like how I didn't do one assignment or test on my own my last year. I literally could not think and felt daily headaches everyday at school or at home. Some days I would go to bed with a headache and severe neckpain only to wake up with it being worse. I felt sick all day long and my girlfriend christinia couldn't understand why I just wanted to sit at home alone in my dark basement . . .

"I thought about suicide quite a bit back then and I never understood what was wrong with me. I never understood [where] the big strong Zac Easter went or why.

"All I know is that I have never been the same."

FIVE

The Coach and the Trainer

I DIDN'T HAVE to be around him for more than a few minutes to realize that Eric Kluver is a Real Football Man. At forty-six, he is thick, muscular, and barrel-chested. His brown hair is closely cropped in a buzz cut, and his small, steel-blue, close-set eyes cast a penetrating gaze. At the end of summer, Kluver's face and neck are beet-red like a farmer's. He's spent the first part of the summer outside running his landscaping business, and the second part outside coaching football. He's sitting in his red-brick office in the bowels of Indianola High School. A television is cued up with football tape. A lonely, sunken plaid couch sits in the corner. A whistle hangs from his neck.

If you're a parent whose son wants to play football, this is the type of man you want to be his coach. He yells—of course he yells; this is football, for God's sake—but his idle position is that of a nurturing coach and a decent man. He is a father figure who, after he rants at halftime about how the defense needs to maintain focus and not commit stupid infractions that result in penalties, downshifts to a soothing tone and tells his players how proud he is of them. When he talks about why he loves coaching, he doesn't focus on the big wins or the state titles because in a place like Indianola, which has always played bigger and stronger schools, there aren't

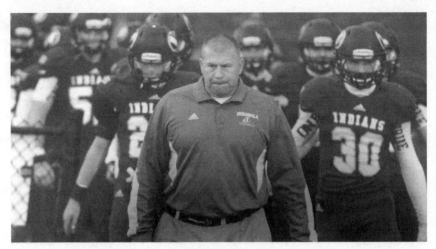

Eric Kluver believes football is the best sport to create strong male leaders of high character.

an overwhelming number of big wins, and there certainly aren't any state titles. Instead, he talks about football as the perfect sport to teach young men about life.

"I don't know if there's another sport that prepares you for life like the game of football," Kluver tells me in his office. "It's the ultimate team sport. You can be a heckuva player, but if you're not on all cylinders as a team, you're probably not going to be successful. The qualities that you learn from the game of football you'll take with you for the rest of your life. Being on time. Responsibility, discipline, work ethic, being loyal, being a good communicator and a great teammate. Those are all things you have to use later in life. That's why I feel that playing the game of football, it's just irreplaceable."

These words may seem like the clichés you'd hear from any Real Football Man, someone who considers his football-playing years the best of his life and who stays around the game so he can rekindle the excitement from his own glory days. Yet Kluver's full-throated endorsement of football comes with a deep moral ambivalence. He is simultaneously in a lifelong love affair with the sport while being racked by guilt about what he's experienced in the sport. Because on three separate occasions, Kluver has experienced the absolute worst that can come out of football. He struggles with his own role in it, specifically in Zac Easter's death.

Listen to Kluver's guilt: "There's a lot of people out there: 'I can't believe they allowed this! These terrible coaches and athletic directors! How can you let this happen?' Stuff like that. But, we just didn't know. That was five years ago. We didn't know! He was a tough kid. His dad was on the staff. He obviously lied about how he was feeling with all the concussions."

Kluver pauses and collects his thoughts. He's not crying. Real Football Men do not cry. But his voice gets quiet, thoughtful, emotional. "We called it 'dinged up.' But it wasn't like Zac was staggering around all the time. That's the shocking part now, after everything has unfolded. Because you do think, 'How could I have missed this? It was so obvious!' But in reality, it really wasn't.

"I truly, honestly didn't know what was happening to him. I think I'm able to cope with it easier because I didn't know. Because none of us knew. But yet the guilt is there. Because we *shoulda* known. I'll be a better coach because of that. We can't let this ever happen again."

For Americans who aren't obsessed with football, the equation is simple: The sport is, by its very nature, dangerous; young people are sustaining life-changing injuries in numbers that are too high for our society to stomach; our society must stop its endorsement of this activity, especially among our youth. Crystal clear. But for a Real Football Man like Kluver, the equation is much more complicated because all things that help turn a boy into a man must come with some element of risk. Yes, the sport must be made safer, both for the players' safety and for the sport's survival. But he worries about going too far, and risking what he sees as the essence of the best sport to help form a man. The sport that has wrought so much bad has also brought even more good. For Kluver, saving football is of vital importance.

The concussion crisis has upended high school football as much as it's upended the NFL. The speed with which high school students are shying away from football has increased in recent years as football's concussion crisis has been recognized as something that's not just affecting fifteen-year NFL veterans. Since its peak in 2008–09, participation in eleven-player tackle football has declined nearly 10 percent among American high school boys, according to the National Federation of State High School Associations (NFHS). Nearly thirty-one thousand fewer American high school boys played eleven-player tackle football during the 2018–19 school year than the year before, according to data from the NFHS. That's a 3 percent drop in participation in just one year.

But let's not kid ourselves: A 10 percent drop is significant, and it meant that 106,290 fewer high school boys played football in 2018 compared with 2008, but that still means more than one million American high school boys played football in 2018. That's nearly double the next-closest sport among boys: 605,354 boys participated in outdoor track and field, 540,769 played basketball, 482,740 played baseball, and 459,077 played soccer. Backers of high school football, even the ones like Myles Easter Sr. who bemoan the sissification of the sport, acknowledge that the sport's future centers on containing the concussion crisis. That's why Eric Kluver has turned over all the authority on whether a player reenters a game or a practice after a big hit from the coaching staff to the trainer. It's why Kluver, in the first season after Zac Easter's death, started teaching a rugby-like style of tackling that involves taking the head out of the impact of the tackle. It's why Kluver has outfitted the entire team with Guardian Caps, a soft-shell protective cover that slides over football helmets. His team now wears these in practice. They look a bit goofy, as if each player is wearing a black mushroom on top of his helmet, but Kluver thinks they work, softening the impact of hits to the head.

The sport's concussion crisis is also why he's changed his mentality as a coach.

"I would say I'm an old-school coach. But boy, I sure err on the safe side now. I can't always say I did that," Kluver admits. "I have some former players on our staff. They'll be like, 'What?'" They were shocked that practice was already over. "'We used to run forever, practice forever! I can't believe how easy these guys got it!' But when you go through some tragedy, it really is an eye-opener."

Kluver spent his early years on an acreage in rural Iowa. With two older brothers and one younger, any ball became a source of entertainment. By the time the family moved to Ankeny when Kluver was in fifth grade, to the same hulking suburban school district that Zac Easter and his teammates would so despise a generation later, the Kluver family's focus had turned exclusively to football. Ankeny was lingering between being a small town amidst the farm fields and a growing suburb in the orbit of Des Moines. Kluver and his family dove into the football traditions that defined Ankeny's Friday nights in the fall. What struck Kluver even then was that the younger boys looked up to the high school players as heroes, and yet these same boys were literally the boys next door: friends of the family, or fellow congregants at church, or cashiers at the gas station. Football in small-town Iowa was an intimate spectacle.

Kluver's oldest brother starred in high school and walked on at the University of Iowa, where he played center. Another brother was a long snapper at Iowa State University in Ames. By the time Kluver entered high school in the late 1980s, the only thing he wanted was to be the next Kluver in line to play football for their community. It was not unlike the feeling the three Easter brothers would have a generation later in Indianola. Kluver played linebacker, like Zac, and like his future player, Kluver loved to hit hard.

The team was called the Ankeny Hawks, and the coaches had a special tradition: For a big hit—those special big hits that come only a few times a season, when you absolutely obliterate an opponent, and the players and the crowd roar in unison—the coaches would hand out a BAD HAWK T-shirt during the Monday-morning meeting after a game. It was Kluver's goal during his high school football career to get one of those BAD HAWK shirts. His senior year, Kluver's team was playing Fort Dodge, a small city in the north-central part of the state. On one particular play, the ball was snapped and Kluver stunted, switching roles with a defensive teammate to confuse the blockers. He ripped right past the blockers and sprinted into the backfield with a full head of steam. He hit the running back, who was much bigger than Kluver, hard enough to lift both of his legs off the ground. Kluver wrapped him up and slammed him into the turf. The next Monday morning, the coaches held the team meeting, and Kluver was presented with a BAD HAWK for that hit. Nearly thirty years later, Kluver still speaks of that moment with great excitement, one of those small but meaningful snapshots that stick with you for life: "It's not one of those shirts you use as a rag. It's pretty sacred." Those BIG HAMMER T-shirts that Kluver gave out when he later became a coach are an homage to the BAD HAWK T-shirts from his own high school career.

That same senior season brought Kluver's first football tragedy. It was the summer of 1990. One of Kluver's closest friends,
Matt Hanke, who was a year behind him in school, had been in
a car accident earlier that summer, so he missed the first several
weeks of football practice. He was released by his doctors to play
right before the team's annual intrasquad scrimmage. The play that
caused Hanke to collapse wasn't particularly remarkable. Kluver
doesn't remember what exactly happened, just some sort of hit to
the head. But Kluver vividly recalls what occurred moments after,
when he was standing over his friend on the field.

"He's groaning, his eyes are rolled back," Kluver remembers.
"You're in high school. You think you're invincible. We thought
he was a big, tough, strong kid, so everything would be all right.
[So] we all took our time to get down to the hospital. We didn't
understand the severity of the injury. It became very obvious when
we walked into the emergency room and saw the family."

Hanke had suffered a subdural hematoma. After the hit to
the head, blood rapidly filled the area between his brain and the
dura, the sheath-like membrane that covers the brain. The pool-
ing blood compressed his brain tissue. By the time his teammates
arrived at the hospital, Hanke was sedated and in a coma. Doctors
sliced out part of his skull to relieve the pressure. Kluver's friend
did not die immediately, and that alone was considered a medical
success, given the extent of his injury. Kluver and a small group
of guys from the football team spent much of the rest of the
school year at Hanke's side in the hospital, playing cards, doing
homework, just being present with their friend. After the injury,
Hanke's life completely changed. He got around in a wheelchair.
He permanently moved into a rehabilitation facility in Waterloo,
two hours northeast of his family's Ankeny home. It took him

five more years to graduate from high school. He died in 2007, at age thirty-three.

Kluver takes a deep breath and shakes his head.

"It almost makes me sick to keep doing what I'm doing," he tells me. He's spent many nights grappling with the downsides of the game he loves so deeply. So much good comes from football, but there can be plenty of bad as well. He doesn't want to put young lives at risk by sending the youths out on a football field, but he also doesn't believe American boys ought to be coddled in Bubble Wrap, protected from every danger out there. At some point, you must live life, and for Kluver, football is an enormous part of life, one of the biggest parts.

When Kluver stood over Zac Easter's casket more than a quarter century after his high school friend's brain injury on the football field, he felt a special kind of grief. Kluver loves all his players, but this wasn't just any player in the casket. This was Zac Easter, the son of Kluver's top assistant. Kluver knew the brain is a complicated thing, and that there were plenty of factors that led to Zac's death—other concussions suffered outside of football, mental illness, drinking and drug use—but certainly, football played a significant part. And there was a chicken-and-egg question here: Was Zac going to struggle no matter what with mental illness and substance abuse, or did football set all those struggles in motion? Kluver could explain away Hanke's death as an accident, a freak occurrence that could have happened on a football field or on a soccer field or in a car wreck or while riding a bike down the street. But Zac's death? This was no accident. This was football.

Maybe this was the universe telling Kluver that he should walk away from the sport.

But . . .

It's complicated.

"I truly believe what I'm doing is benefiting young men to become better people," Kluver says. "They're developing qualities they're going to need in life. I've gained so much from football. It made me a man. I'd hate to see it go away. In life, you're going to go through a lot of tough situations, no different than a football game. Some people say that's not a good comparison. But truly: How are you going to react to adversity in your life? Are you going to quit? Give up? Or fight forward and make the most of it?"

Kluver's views are representative of a wide swath of American males whose definition of manhood is in large part formed by football. The ideal man is a disciplined part of a team, takes coaching and does not complain, puts his head down and does the hard work. The Easter mentality, in other words. But adherents of this Easter mentality believe there's a part of progressive modern-day America that is using the current concern around concussions and CTE to attack not just the sport of football but the very archetype of the American male that football creates and represents. It's not just that concussions are bad and should be reduced—who would disagree with that premise? Instead, it's that this Easter mentality, this ideal of the American man, has been rebranded by progressives as "toxic masculinity." That's why people like Kluver believe it's not just football that's under attack these days. It's their version of manhood that's in the crosshairs: the strong, tough, stoic type of American male that helped build this country.

"Those deaths, those injuries, they put things in perspective in a hurry—in a *hurry*," Kluver says. "There's definitely been times where I've said, 'Is this worth it?' The game of football helped me get through all those injuries and deaths, and yet the game of football also caused them. But I also know those guys wouldn't have had it any other way, that they loved football that much."

Perhaps it's because he truly believes the good that comes from football outweighs the bad. Or perhaps it's because Kluver is, like a vast chunk of Americans, addicted to the sport of football, and he can't imagine football going away, can't imagine life without football. Kluver knows one thing: Despite all these tragedies, football is, in the most definitive way possible, worth it.

A HALF HOUR before kickoff, the team retreats to its locker room of Indianola High School's new $6 million athletic complex, built a few years after Levi, the last of the football-playing Easter boys, graduated in 2011. The players sit quietly, as if in church pews. Kluver paces behind them. The coach's voice is quiet, almost prayerful, as he calls for the boys to focus: "Getting dialed in, getting dialed in. Ready to turn it loose now. Fast start, fast start." The players form a circle and take a knee, helmets resting on the ground. For sixty seconds, not a word. It's quiet enough in here that you can hear the soundtrack from the other side of the door, conjuring these scenes from a fall Friday night in America's heartland: parents holding giant Fathead posters of high school players, cheerleaders with fresh layers of sparkly lip gloss chanting next to students with chests painted in school colors, a public address announcer introducing middle-school football players to the fans filling the grandstands as "our FUTURE Indianola Indians!"

Then, the varsity players start banging their helmets on the cement floor, quiet at first, louder, then reaching a crescendo. Kluver's persona shifts, from meditating minister to army general. The coach peers through the crack in the double doors. "Here we go, boys," he says. Time to storm Normandy. The doors fly open: The click of spikes on cement. Middle schoolers lined up, wide-eyed, giving high fives as players stride past. Fireworks shooting into the sky. And later, cannon blasts after every Indianola touchdown, an assistant coach (perhaps a bit too into the moment) instructing his defense to "KILLKILLKILL!," the sweeping sensation of seventy-some teenage boys all rooting for the same thing. In these moments, there is nothing bigger than football, no more important thing in the entire world.

Of course we're a nation addicted to football.

How can you *not* get addicted to this feeling?

And what would be lost if football—the sport Eric Kluver believes turns boys into men, that has helped turn our country into what it is today—is softened in the name of safety, and of treating what some see as a harmful national addiction?

The scope of our addiction to football and its cathartic form of violence is mind-boggling. The NFL made $15 billion in revenue in 2018 and has a stated goal of reaching $25 billion in annual revenue by 2027. *Forbes* in 2019 ranked twenty-six NFL franchises as among the fifty most valuable sports franchises in the world. The Dallas Cowboys, worth $5 billion, topped the list as the world's most valuable sports franchise. The eight most-watched television broadcasts in American history have been Super Bowls. College football, often looked at as the minor-league feeder to the NFL, is also a cash cow. ESPN's fee for broadcast rights to the College Football Playoff for twelve years, starting with the 2014 season, comes to $87 million for *each game*. Even the pretend versions of American football have become national obsessions; *Madden NFL* is one of the best-selling video game franchises of all time, having sold more than 130 million copies, and some 75 million Americans play fantasy football, by far the most popular sport in the $18 billion fantasy sports industry.

Football means much more to Americans than just a way to spend a few hours on a weekend afternoon. The sport that was called The Great God Football nearly a century ago has morphed into an American football-industrial complex that stands unrivaled in the history of sport. And while our national addiction is most apparent on Saturdays and Sundays, in the cathedrals to football that are NFL and collegiate stadiums, the seeds for this addiction are planted on Friday nights in late summer and fall, when one million high school boys get their first real taste of football glory, and when America's full-fledged addiction to this sport is at its most relatable, its most boy-next-door.

There are plenty of big sociological conclusions about America that we can come to through our football addiction. In his 1993 book *Reading Football: How the Popular Press Created an American Spectacle*, Michael Oriard described the plurality of meanings of football in America, which can be extrapolated into an explanation of why our national sport crosses every social, economic, and ethnic barrier: "Football is important to the corporate America that leases luxury boxes at NFL stadiums; to the religious right that proselytizes through such groups as the Fellowship for Christian Athletes and Athletes in Action; to ghetto blacks and coal miners' sons in Pennsylvania dreaming of escape into American success; to southerners for whom football is tied to long traditions of honor in blood sports; to middle-class white boys in high schools throughout the country simply looking for social acceptance and relief from unleashed hormones; to their fathers dreaming of glory they once or never had, driving their sons to prove, as Don DeLillo memorably put it in his novel *End Zone*, that the seed has not been impoverished."

Perhaps the biggest sociological conclusion to be drawn from our football addiction is this: that the primal feeling it illuminates is by no means unique to America. In fact, the attraction humans have had toward these spectacles of mostly controlled violence has been present since . . . well, since the first instances of humanity playing sports. The words of George Orwell about what spectator sports conjure in humanity ring especially true in football, when he writes of the "sadistic pleasure in witnessing violence." "Games were built up into a heavily financed activity, capable of attracting vast crowds and rousing savage passions, and the infection spread from country to country," Orwell wrote. "It is the most violently combative sports, football and boxing, that have spread the widest."

The most popular spectator sports have always been violent, noted R. Todd Jewell in his academic book, *Violence and Aggression in Sporting Contests: Economics, History and Policy.* Violence adds drama and risk. Studies have researched the types of sports that men and women most viscerally respond to, and while women show the greatest enjoyment from watching—as Jewell noted—"elegant stylistic sports" like gymnastics, for men it's always been the more violent the better. "For men, excitement increased when violence was exhibited in athletic forms," Jewell wrote of one study's results. It's a way for sports spectators to experience the catharsis of violence vicariously, and from the safety of their viewing spot in the grandstands or on their couch. For many men, it seems, they can fully appreciate the beauty of an athletic maneuver only if the possibility of a violent and disruptive collision is right around the corner.

In the first recorded Olympic Games in ancient Greece in 776 BC, there was only one sport: the footrace. But it should come as no surprise that boxing and wrestling were soon added, as well as other sports that included the possibility of death, like chariot racing. "Since the beginning of time, humans have had types of play fighting—fighting for the pleasure of fighting rather than for attack," said Dominic Malcolm, a sports sociologist at England's Loughborough University and the editor of the *International Review for the Sociology of Sport*. Paleolithic cave paintings from more than fifteen thousand years ago in France may depict sprinting and wrestling, while Mongolian cave paintings dating back some nine thousand years show crowds of spectators surrounding a wrestling match. Wrestling is the only sport mentioned in the Bible. Historians guess that the earliest version of sport came as a form of military training, to determine whether males would be useful for military service.

The combat sport that was most popular in ancient Greece was called pankration, a warrior-like contest with few rules. The aim was to either get your opponent to give up or to kill him. The ancient Greeks discovered exactly how useful training in combat sports could be for their military after the Battle of Marathon in 490 BC, in which much of the fighting was hand-to-hand, according to classicist Michael B. Poliakoff. In ancient Rome, gladiator combat pitted armed men, typically either slaves or criminals, against one another or against wild animals like lions, bears, elephants, tigers, crocodiles, and hippopotamuses. The gladiatorial fights between humans and wild beasts were called *venatio*, and thousands of animals would be slaughtered during a single day's competition. The risks of gladiatorial combat, such as severe injuries or death, were offset somewhat by the opportunity for money and heroism.

In Central America, the Mayans played a racquetball-like game known as *pokolpok*; the sport simulated battle, and the losers were sacrificed to the gods. The Native Americans of North America started playing a version of lacrosse some twenty-five hundred years ago; the sport was a religious ritual that simulated war, and games would involve hundreds of players and last for days. The word that the Onondaga tribe of northeastern North America used for its antecedent to lacrosse was *dehuntshigwa'es*, or "little war." In ancient Egypt, the so-called sport of fisherman jousting involved small boats with a handful of competitors who tried to knock one another into the water. Since swimming wasn't something ancient Egyptians were particularly proficient in, competitions often ended in drownings. The medieval times of Europe brought the armored knight as the most prominent heavy cavalry warrior, and with that rose the violent sport of jousting.

Over the past century, a frequent debate among anthropologists is whether violence, and by extension the enduring popularity of violent sports, is an innate part of human nature or something that's learned through society. In other words: Is violence in our DNA? Anthropologists posit two theories on the origin of humans' instinct toward aggression and war, a relationship that can be extended to violent sports. Essentially, it's a nature-versus-nurture argument. One is the "drive discharge" model, which argues that individual humans have an innate drive toward aggression and violence that generates an internal tension. That tension can be relieved through the discharge of violence. This theory argues that aggressive behavior finds an outlet one way or another. This sort of innate predilection toward violence (and thus toward violent sports) is related to the "killer ape hypothesis," which theorizes that war and interpersonal aggression were the primary forces behind humans evolving from apes. You could think of the drive discharge model as the "boys will be boys" interpretation. In this theory, violent sports help assuage humans' natural instinct toward violence, so the presence of violent sports can actually mean a less violent society. This is the theory that Sigmund Freud ascribed to; he called sport a "substitute discharge." "Warlike sports serve to discharge accumulated aggressive tension and therefore act as alternative channels to war, making it less likely," explained Richard G. Sipes in his academic paper, "War, Sports and Aggression: An Empirical Test of Two Rival Theories."

The other argument is the "culture pattern" model, which suggests that individual violent, aggressive behavior is primarily learned through society. According to this theory, the presence of violent sports in a society actually increases that society's inclinations toward war. The inverse would also be true: "The probability of war can be reduced, according to this model, by decreasing the incidence of combative sports and other behavior similar to warfare," Sipes asserted in his paper for the academic journal *American Anthropologist*. While sociologists and anthropologists of Freud's generation generally hewed to the theory that violence is innate, the past few generations of sociologists and anthropologists have convened over the idea that a human being learns to glorify violence through society. The modern theory posits that societies with a predilection toward violent sports like football and boxing end up being more violent and warlike than societies that don't have a preference for violent sports. This suggests aggressive sports actually increase the overall violence in our society instead of just providing us with a release for the innate violent tendencies already inside us. This is obviously very theoretical. But Sipes offered evidence for how a violent culture can be connected to violent sports; he found that football spectatorship increased substantially during World War II, the Korean War, and the Vietnam War, while spectatorship of the nonviolent sport of baseball dropped during each of those conflicts only to recover afterward.

No matter which theory is correct, there certainly is something about America that makes our country especially attracted to a sport that's based on violent collisions as a core principle. Our nation was birthed through violence: against the Native American population by the first European settlers, against Africans brought to the colonies as slaves, and then against the British during the Revolutionary War. Our country spends roughly the same amount annually on its military, some $650 billion, as the next eight countries combined, according to a 2019 report by the Stockholm International Peace Research Institute. Despite considering ourselves an orderly, civilized people, violence is now and always has been a central part of American life. A 2018 study by the Institute for Health Metrics and Evaluation, affiliated with the University of Washington in Seattle, indicated that only Brazil had more firearm-related deaths in 2016 than the 37,200 in the United States. The Global Peace Index 2019 ranks 163 countries by how dangerous they are, and the United States ranks as the thirty-fifth most dangerous country in the world. But it's the fourth most dangerous country in the Western hemisphere; only Colombia, Venezuela, and Mexico are considered more dangerous. (Countries less dangerous than the United States include Honduras, Guatemala, and El Salvador.) And that thirst for violence extends to sport. There's something sadistic about the fact that our national sport, the game that Americans most often play together and watch together, is one in which we take pleasure in people hurting other people.

All this can be read as further reason to eradicate the violence from football. Since humans have evolved beyond our early savagery, shouldn't our sports evolve beyond their savageries as well? Haven't we, as a civilization that's learned how to fly, that's traveled to the moon, that's connected an entire world through the Internet—haven't we become, well, *better than that*?

And yet: If human nature is to be violent, how cautious must we be about watering down the sport? Yes, the health of athletes—specifically of high school and middle school athletes who won't be going on to pro careers, and specifically the health of their brains—is of the utmost importance. But what is lost if football becomes a far less violent sport? Is the direction America's foremost sport is heading something that could make the United States a lesser, weaker nation? Or is America better off to protect our brains at all costs? It's a variation of the question that Eric Kluver has been wrestling with: What is lost when football becomes a safer—or, some would say, a *softer*—sport?

"You do want your players to be tough and disciplined and work through adversity," Kluver said. "You're going to be hurt. But injuries are a different story. A generation ago, playing through injuries, that's what you were supposed to do. That was football. It's different today. Especially with the brain. It's such a delicate part of the body. It's different than a finger, an elbow, a shoulder. There's a lot more caution now in the game of football, and there needs to be."

But not too much caution. That's the beauty of football—that like in life, you have to navigate potential dangers around every corner. Sure, the football tragedies Kluver has experienced have softened him up. But he still thinks it's the greatest game ever invented, and he still thinks that it's the best sport at teaching boys the character traits—responsibility and discipline, teamwork and communication—that it takes to turn them into productive young men. For Kluver, the bottom line is this: Football's physicality, its endemic violence, is an unavoidable part of the sport's allure and its virtue.

"I can't make it bulletproof," Kluver said. "There's going to be collisions. Athletes are becoming stronger, faster, more explosive, even at the lowest of levels, and especially through high school. Kids are so much bigger and stronger and faster than even twenty-five years ago when I was playing. Ultimately, I just know that the good that comes from football outweighs the bad."

Sue Wilson is tall and athletic, with long brown hair that becomes gold tinted in summer. She has a slight gap between her front teeth, and pretty blue eyes that betray the deep wells of empathy that lie within. But do not confuse Wilson's empathy for weakness. This mother of two hockey-playing girls is as tough as they come, an athlete who had battled through her own litany of injuries as a competitive downhill skier while she was growing up in Minnesota. Going through rounds and rounds of painful physical therapy to recover from her knee injuries is what first got her interested in athletic training, which wasn't a popular career choice at that time; Wilson was one of seven students in her program. She got her degree in 2001 from Simpson College in Indianola, which was where she met her future husband, a soccer player who became a youth soccer coach. That was also where she first encountered a gruff football coach named Myles Easter. Wilson needed all the toughness she could muster when, in 2005, she was hired as the athletic trainer at Indianola High School. Her primary responsibility was caring for the dings and dents of the football players. That first team she attended to was small compared with those of other schools in the conference; there were thirty-three players that year, while the bigger schools in the Des Moines suburbs often had twice that. Six of the players had to play both offense and defense—Ironman football, which harked back to the way the game used to be played.

Wilson was hired to protect these athletes, but being hired is different than being *wanted*. And at first, Wilson was most definitely not wanted. She'd often have to answer questions from coaches like Myles Easter: "Is that guy really hurt?" She was the first full-time athletic trainer in the school's history, and one of her main focuses, especially for football, was concussions. She often felt cast in the role of Mrs. No: the willful, persistent woman who was standing on the sidelines for the most manly of sports, telling players whose bodies appeared perfectly healthy that an injury they couldn't see—a mysterious, nebulous injury inside their brains—was going to keep them out of a football game. "I spent the first ten years of my career taking helmets away from kids," Wilson said.

Again and again, she'd hear the same words from a coach when she pulled a player out of a game for a suspected concussion: "You know how many times I hit my head when I played? This is ridiculous!" Parents would pull her aside: "Put him back in," they'd say about their son, who Wilson suspected had a concussion. But Wilson has thick skin, so she held on to the helmet, even if there were only small lingering signs of a concussion. "That's my job, not yours," Wilson would tell the dissenters.

An injury to the brain is not like a broken arm; there's guesswork involved in diagnosing a concussion, especially in the moments after it happens. Wilson always guessed with caution. "At the end of the day, the coaches go home and they're upset about the game and how they performed or didn't perform," Wilson told me. "At the end of the day, I go home and think to myself, 'Is that kid going to cramp?' 'Is he on the verge of heat exhaustion and we didn't deal with it right?' 'Is this kid going to start vomiting at midnight tonight because of a head injury?' If I go home thinking whether I should have sent a kid to a hospital, that's a long night for me."

One particular memory from her first year as Indianola High School's trainer stands out. There was a player, who today is

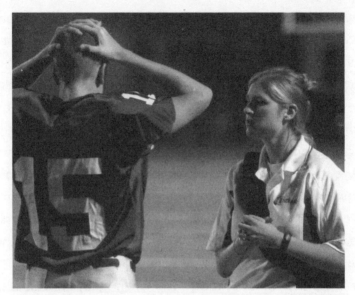

*Sue Wilson was an unwanted presence: The woman who
would tell players to sit out for fear of concussion.*

an emergency room doctor in Minnesota, who was a star wide
receiver and team captain. He took a hit to the head and looked
discombobulated. *An obvious concussion*, Wilson thought. So she
told him he couldn't go back in. "No way," Wilson said. But when
Wilson's attention was elsewhere, the player ran back onto the field
for a play. He appeared woozy and out of it. When he came back
off the field after the play, Wilson watched as he lowered his head
into his hands.

"What's up?" she asked him.

"I'm fine, I'm fine," he replied.

She looked at his eyes. They looked glassy and unable to focus.

"You're done," Wilson told him. "Give me your helmet."

This was Wilson making her first big stand. The crowd was
watching her.

"Fuck you," the player said. He threw his mouthguard at her. The rest of the game, he sat on the sidelines, glaring at her as she clutched his helmet.

"I walked up to Coach Kluver," Wilson recalled, "and I said, 'He's done, and I've got his helmet. So if he ends up back in this game and gets hurt, that's all on you.'" Parents and fans murmured their disapproval. This was a time when there wasn't a standard protocol for a potentially concussed player—the NFL didn't introduce its concussion assessment guidelines until 2013. In the stands, a local doctor walked up to the school's athletic director. "Why does *she* have the authority to take helmets away?" the doctor asked. The next day, the athletic director called her, wondering whether she was actually qualified to take a player's helmet away, to take a team captain out of the game because of a nebulous head injury.

A player telling Wilson to go fuck herself was not exactly out of the ordinary her first few years as Indianola's athletic trainer. Nor was her being doubted by the team's coaches. One of the biggest doubters was Myles Easter, Zac's father. She'd known him for a decade, since he was coaching at Simpson College and she was a student studying to be an athletic trainer, so she felt like she could be blunt with him. "When I'd hold a person out, he'd say, 'I don't know what the problem is. I've probably had eight or nine concussions from playing football and I'm fine. I don't understand why they can't come in and play.' And I'd say, 'That's my job, not yours.' He'd just walk away." Zac was the same way. Wilson did a baseline cognitive test at the beginning of each season so she could better determine if a player had a concussion later in the season. In that baseline test, she asked each player to say the months of the year backward. Her first memory of Zac was during this baseline test his freshman year. "Where do I start?" he said. Sue paused: "Well, December, if you're doing them backwards." He was indignant. Yes, he was able to, but he was also stubborn, and he just didn't want to do this concussion test. "I don't even know the month now," he said. "I just know it's football time." *An Easter*, Wilson thought. *Of course this is an Easter.*

"The first three years were horrendous," Wilson recalled about the time when she was constantly second-guessed. "And then we had Joey Goodale and his huge head injury."

Joey Goodale was the second of the three big football tragedies that Eric Kluver has experienced in his football career. Joey was a joyful sophomore at Indianola High School, in the same class (and on the same football team) as Levi Easter, Zac's younger brother. Joey was the type of kid who was always the life of the party; he was friends with Zac Easter and a kindred spirit on the football field. Like Zac, Joey was a middle brother with something to prove. Sports were central to his identity: Baseball, wrestling, and most of all, football. Joey had always been a big kid. He was almost eleven pounds when he was born.

"He came out as a football player," said his mother, Dawn Goodale. The sport came naturally to him. His dad had played football in high school and college. All in the family were fans of the Notre Dame Fighting Irish and the Iowa Hawkeyes. Joey started playing youth football in grade school, and he was so excited to finally get into a Pop Warner league, the biggest youth football organization in the United States, and put on the pads. As an offensive lineman and a defensive end, Joey loved to throw his body into the fray. He'd had a couple of concussions before high school, but he wanted to keep playing football. His mom didn't like the idea. She thought about not letting him play in high school.

But who was she to get in the way of her teenage son's football dreams?

It was a normal football play during a normal football practice, a Tuesday night in August 2008, not long after school started and not long before the team's first game of the season. They were working on kickoff returns. Joey was on the front line of blockers for the side that was returning the kickoff. The kicker accidentally popped the ball up, a short kick, so all the players were running toward one another. Joey was hit and fell backward. He smacked the back of his head on the ground. "Joey, you all right?" someone shouted. "Good, coach!" Joey replied, and then ran back to the huddle.

A couple of minutes later, Joey took another hit to the head. Again, nothing remarkable. But this time, Joey walked toward Sue on the sidelines. "Sue, I just feel weird," he said.

"OK, let's take your helmet off," Sue told him.

He said his legs felt wobbly. She told him to sit down. She looked into eyes. His pupils blew out. Then, his legs gave out, and he fell into Wilson's arms before collapsing to the turf. "We gotta call 911!" Wilson yelled to Kluver. Inside his skull, Joey's brain was bleeding, just like Kluver's friend Matt Hanke's had some two decades before. Standing over Joey on the field, Kluver's mind flashed back.

Joey was in the midst of a full-blown seizure. His whole body went rigid. Out of his mouth came a terrifying groaning noise. Wilson lay next to him and spoke directly into his ears: "Stay with me, Joe, stay with me." She rubbed his sternum. Wilson cut off his jersey and pads just in case the EMTs needed to use a defibrillator. It was twelve or thirteen minutes before the ambulance showed up. The EMTs put Joey on a stretcher. The ambulance idled. The EMTs

weren't going fast enough for Wilson: "Why aren't you guys moving? His brain is bleeding! He's not going to come out of it until
they drill a hole in his skull!"

Kluver got in the back of the ambulance. Joey was breathing
but unconscious. The EMTs intubated him to ease his breathing.
The ambulance raced up and down the hills of US Highway 69,
past the grain silos, past the miles of farmland and forest, and then
the miles of strip malls and chain restaurants, sprinting toward the
emergency room at Blank Children's Hospital in Des Moines. The
entire drive, Kluver thought Joey was going to die. In Indianola,
Wilson, who was still at practice, kept calling Joey's mother, but
her phone was off. His dad was on a golf course and couldn't be
reached. Wilson sent an assistant superintendent to pick up Joey's
mother and drive her to the hospital.

Back on the field, nobody knew what to do: A teenage boy had
just collapsed on the field, and the head coach had jumped into
the ambulance headed to the hospital. So the defensive coordinator, Myles Easter Sr., piped up with a plan: They would continue
the practice. They had a game coming up. Plus, they had to get the
boys' minds moving, not staying focused on Joey. Fifteen minutes
after the ambulance had left, Zac Easter's knee got clipped on a
play, and he hobbled off to the sideline with a strained medial col-
lateral ligament. It would keep Zac, then a junior, out of practice
for a few days.

By 7:00 p.m., the entire football team and the players' parents—more than a hundred people in all, including Zac Easter
and his father—had gathered in the waiting room at the hospital.
Doctors explained to Joey's family that he had severed a vein that
runs through the brain, and it was bleeding. Surgeons removed a
flap of bone from the fifteen-year-old's skull to relieve the pressure.

The surgeon explained the uncertainty: "He could walk out of here tomorrow, he could be here for months, he could die tonight." A chaplain prayed with the family.

For the next three weeks, Joey remained in a coma in the intensive care unit. He developed pneumonia, so doctors put in a tracheostomy tube. Almost every afternoon, Wilson and Kluver made the drive from Indianola to Des Moines to visit Joey and his family in the hospital. His head was swollen. They prayed over him as they watched his body shed weight. After three weeks, like in a movie, Joey suddenly woke up from the coma. His mother was at his bedside. He could talk, but not well, so he gave his mom a thumbs-up.

The upcoming years would be difficult for Joey. He learned to speak again in speech therapy. His food came to him through an IV in his nose until he learned how to swallow properly. He went through physical therapy and occupational therapy. He returned to school in November with a one-on-one associate accompanying him. His short-term memory was terrible, his cognition not nearly what it had been. His personality changed in a way that many people's personalities do after traumatic brain injuries. He became much more honest, almost to a fault, as if he had zero social filter. He developed a love-hate relationship with football; he still looked back fondly on his years playing the sport, and yet he recognized this was the sport that nearly killed him. For years, he struggled with alcohol and drugs, saying those were the only things that made him feel normal. Some days, he'd be drunk by noon. His parents put him in an in-patient Christian-based home for teens and adults struggling with substance abuse. He didn't go to college even though his two brothers went to elite private colleges.

In time, Joey found his own path. He got a part-time job at the local Fareway grocery store, unloading trucks starting at 5:00 a.m.

These days, he works out three days a week. He reads Christian devotionals in the morning and at night. He goes to church weekly, and to Christian youth group meetings at Simpson College.

But when he was in the coma, his parents didn't know what his new normal might someday look like. First, they just wanted him to live.

While Joey was still in the coma, the Indianola High School football team took a vote. The players wanted to do something meaningful for their teammate. They decided to recognize Joey for his toughness on the football field as well as his toughness as he recovered from the injury. Even though he wasn't conscious, they hoped their little gesture would be appreciated, and perhaps give him a small mental boost. Zac Easter and another teammate drove up to Des Moines after a football practice one evening and went into Joey's hospital room. Zac presented him with one of the coveted Indianola football T-shirts: BIG HAMMER.

SIX

The Roller Coaster

"I WANT TO tell my own life story," Zac Easter typed, "just in case something ever happens to me and I'd rather tell my own story through my eyes about my secret struggle before anyone tries to tell my story like nothing was wrong. I swear on everything in my life that I am telling the truth and telling my life story exactly as I remember it because for me, I can finally take off my mask I wear every day. I realize that some of this might be shocking for some of you reading this because I am an expert at waking up every day and putting on my fake mask to do everything I can to not show any weakness, and not let anyone know what I'm actually going through and why I actually do some of the things I do. I was always able to disguise a lot of my actions in the eyes of other people by making it look like I was just extremely motivated or something like that.

"Working out was my only escape when I realized something wsa off with me from the concussions. For years, working out has been the only thing that actually made me feel human again and made me feel less depressed. The only way I knew how to handle my depression and feel good inside was by my on my faith in god, listening to music, lifting, and running. Many people just thought that I was super motivated and determined to be army special forces, but in reality I kept up the super muscle image to look tough on the outside when I was really crying everyday on the inside . . . Obviously this was able to only help for so long before working out stopped taking me to my happy place where I was free of the internal pain. It's hard to hold back tears even now when I think about the times I was feeling so down from depression that I loaded up my .22 rifle or shotgun and put it to my head, and instead talk myself out of out by going for a run in the trails out back and coming inside to lie to my about how I'm such an army badass and how I'm going to be special forces."

IT WAS COLD in the timber.

The Easter men had woken up well before sunrise on December 5, 2009, eaten a hearty breakfast, packed up their firearms, and hopped in the pickup, heading west. Barely a month before, Zac had played in his final high-school football game. The concussion he had suffered in that game would end his sporting career. Wrestling, a sport that's insanely popular in the upper Midwest during the long, windy months of winter on the plains, was no longer a possibility for Zac. Sue Wilson had refused to clear him. But no school trainer could stop him from one of the most joyful experiences of winter for an Easter man: hunting deer with his dad and his brothers.

To get to the family's timber—that same land that had been homesteaded by the boys' great-great-great-great-grandfather, Jacob Stickler, a century and a half before—the Easter men drove up and down the gravel roller coaster that bisects farm fields near their house, onto the pavement, over Interstate 35, past the huge industrial chicken farm, past the white house at the top of the hill where Zac's dad grew up, and right onto Heritage Avenue. The truck's headlights shone in the darkness as the Stringtown

Cemetery, where generations of the Easter family had been buried, appeared on the left. On the right was the big metal gate leading to their property.

The truck bumped over the rocky terrain—plenty of trucks have gotten stuck here on muddier days—and meandered down the hill. The Easter men got out, grabbed their guns, and strode into the timber. Generations of hunters in this family had stalked this land, all the way back to an ancestor who'd participated in Sherman's March to the Sea during the Civil War. The men walked through a clearing and up a wooded hill. To one side were the tall cliffs above the meandering North River and Howerdon Creek, full of carp and catfish. Somewhere nearby was a cave where a World War I veteran, shell-shocked from the war, harmless, but with a spooky glass eye, had once made his home.

By 7:30 a.m., first light had crept over the horizon. The Easter men were strategically spread out through the trees on the side of the hill, connected by cell phones so they could text one another their hunting plans. Zac's older brother, Myles II, had his doubts that they'd find any deer of note that day. He'd spent untold hours here during the bow-hunting season earlier in the fall and never saw a single thing worth a shot. But the other Easter men suspected deer might be running along the ridge of this hill, like they sometimes did. It was minutes after sunrise, which marks the moment when you can legally shoot at deer, when three or four shots rang out of the stillness. They came from the vicinity of where Zac was stationed, three hundred yards or so away from Myles II.

"What'd you hit, Elmer Fudd?" Zac's older brother texted him.

"Just a monster ten-point buck," Zac texted back.

Another text message popped up in Myles II's phone: A picture of the ten-point buck Zac had just slayed. The antler rack was tall

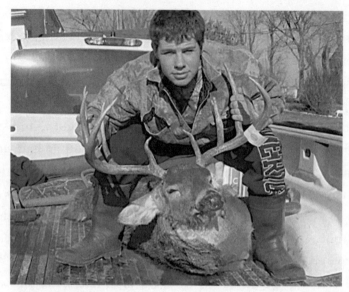

The highlight of Zac's senior year wasn't football.
It was the 10-point buck he bagged in December.

and wide. The deer was huge. The men struggled to pull it down the hill toward their truck. This was a big deal. The family would take this one to a taxidermist, and soon, the neck and head of the buck Zac killed that morning would be mounted on the living room wall, the biggest and most beautiful hunting prize the Easter family had ever bagged, Zac's lifelong trump card over his brothers and even his father.

This was good: A happy moment Zac would remember forever.

The rest of his senior year in high school was the furthest thing from good, and the furthest thing from happy.

"My senior year of high school was the worst," Zac wrote. "I took pro hormones to get absolutely jacked and I don't think the hormones helped with any of the concussions problems either. After my last concussion in high school my life went into the shitter on the inside. Back then I also wasn't very self aware and had no idea that the concussions are what fucked me up. Something changed in me after that last concussion against Ankeny. My depression kicked into full gear and I started having symptoms of anxiety. My emotions have never been the same after the last football concussion either."

Football was over. Soon, so was high school. Whatever the reasons—the head injuries suffered in football, the drinking and partying, the usual self-doubt any teenager experiences when transitioning from the safety of the family home to the uncertainty of the world beyond—Zac felt like a completely different person after high school. His parents didn't notice anything amiss; he just seemed like a regular old eighteen-year-old kid heading off to college. Sure, there were some issues—a little anxiety, a little depression, a little homesickness—but it never seemed like anything more than the normal growing pains of a teenage boy learning to become his own man.

Zac decided to attend Kirkwood Community College's satellite campus in Iowa City, two hours east of his parents' house. His less-than-great grades meant attending the University of Iowa wasn't a possibility at first, but he wanted that real college experience, so he decided to attend this community college near the U of I's campus. Ask any student about the party scene there, and you'll hear stories about the Ped Mall, the Pedestrian Mall in downtown Iowa City, adjacent to campus. It's essentially Disney World for postadolescents, a carnival of debauchery on Friday and Saturday nights when school is in session. (Trust me—I've been there.)

Zac spent plenty of nights striding down the Ped Mall his freshman year, chasing skirts and skirting cops. The community college campus was small, with buildings dedicated to automotive

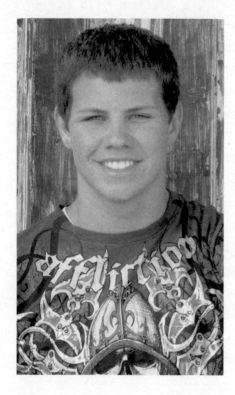

On the surface, it seemed like college-bound Zac had a world of possibilities in front of him.

collision repair and horticulture and swine and beef education. But one of the best parts for Zac was that it was just three miles down the road from Kinnick Stadium. There, nearly seventy thousand fans on fall Saturdays filled the parking lots to tailgate and the bleachers to cheer on the Iowa Hawkeyes football team. The stadium was named after a person who was the Platonic ideal of what a football player aspired to be: Nile Kinnick, the 1939 Heisman Trophy winner (and soon-to-be law student) who Iowans expected would someday become governor, perhaps even president, until he was killed in 1943 as a navy aviator during World War II.

It would have been a dream to take the gridiron wearing the black-and-gold helmets of the Iowa Hawkeyes, but Zac had known for years he was never going to be a Division I football player. He was still steeped in a football mentality, though, so he spent the summer before college filling his body full of those prohormone supplements and pumping iron. Even at his most fit, Zac still noticed his flaws in the mirror before he noticed his brawn. He wanted his body to be ripped, even if punishing workout sessions meant more punishing headaches. At the freshman orientation session before classes started, he ran into a friend from high school, a fellow diehard Green Bay Packers fan from Indianola named Jake Powers, and later that afternoon the two went looking for apartments together. Jake was as workout obsessed as Zac, so once they moved in together, instead of sleeping in beds, they would sleep on couches, set multiple alarms for 4:00 or 4:30 a.m. to make sure they woke up, and go to the gym together for intense training sessions.

Mostly, Zac had a typical college experience: beer and girls and wild nights, with the occasional classes mixed in. One time, Zac's younger brother, Levi, was visiting for the weekend. Zac was napping when there was a fight in the apartment building. During the fight, someone shoved Levi. A friend called Zac to wake him up. Zac jumped out of bed, sprinted down the hall, and tried to destroy the person who'd shoved his brother. Zac busted a door down trying to chase the guy. The cops were called. "I had to grab him, give him a bear hug, and get him out of there," Jake recalled. Another time, Zac and his roommate were out at a party. They found a backpack sitting on a sidewalk, and they picked it up: free backpack! "It was one of our drunker nights," Jake laughed. A kid followed them home, shouting, "That's my bag! That's my bag!" They ignored him. The kid called the cops. Just as the two roommates were about to get on a bus to go back to their apartment, police cars showed up: "Throw the bag on the ground!" one of the officers called out. They were arrested for public intoxication and thrown in the drunk tank with other drunk college kids.

At 5:00 a.m., a fight broke out when one of the drunks peed on someone who was sleeping. Worse still: The next morning, Zac's older brother was playing in a collegiate football game an hour away, and Zac and Jake were supposed to meet Zac's parents at the field before the game. Jake was worried; Zac's dad had been his football coach, and Jake was scared of him. "The whole time we were driving over there, we were like, 'I really don't want to have to face your dad right now,'" Jake said. By the time they made it to the game, it was the middle of the first quarter. Zac's dad was sitting alone at the top of the bleachers, quietly analyzing the game. After a bit, the boys, hungover, worked up the nerve to climb the bleachers and talk to him. "You're not going to believe what happened to us last night," Zac said. They told Myles Sr. the story. "So you guys went to jail?" he said, eyebrows raised. He shook his head. "Hope you learned your lesson." And that was that.

College was fun, but it was the destructive type of fun that masked Zac's bigger issues. He didn't really want to be in college per se. Academics were never his thing. He was there to party, and he was there because he thought that would be the only way he could get back to being the fun, happy-go-lucky Zac Easter from high school: Odie from *Garfield*, that perpetually upbeat dog who was always everybody's friend. But in classes, he felt stupid. He struggled with reading. He struggled writing even a one-page paper. Getting his brain to focus for a single period was a struggle. The depression led to drinking, and the drinking led to more depression, and more depression led to more drinking, and so on.

"Some nights I'd lie in my bed crying wondering what happened to me," he wrote. "I started talking to god and my faith is what carried me though some serious suicidal thoughts."

THERE WAS ONE aspect of college life that gave Zac great pleasure. At the end of his senior year of high school, he filled out paperwork to join the Iowa Army National Guard. He'd always wanted to be in the army, from when he played soldier with friends as a little kid, to when he watched military movies like *Platoon* or *The Deer Hunter* as an older kid, to when he blasted off fireworks and mortars and dynamite in the woods as a near-adult kid. For Zac, the military was like football: a test of being a real man, something that meant he could both indulge and tame his wilder instincts, and ultimately a place that would give him the discipline to make something of himself.

He loved the military. For the next five years, he spent one weekend a month playing soldier on drill weekends and two weeks a year in full-time training. In physical training, Zac was Rambo. "He was a jaw-dropper," said Sgt. Ryan Miller, who was in the same unit as Zac. "It was, 'How in the world can he do this?' He was one of the best soldiers we had." This was no particular surprise to his family members, who knew of Zac's fitness obsessions; after all, he once finished in first place in a national CrossFit competition. When his unit ran, Zac would whip all the other soldiers. His timed two-mile runs came in under twelve minutes. A perfect score for the two-minute push-up test was considered sixty-eight push-ups; Zac would routinely get in the ninetics. He'd get 100 percent in the sit-up test. When the entire company of a hundred or so soldiers did their official physical training test, Miller finished in second place with a score of 280 points. Zac finished in first,

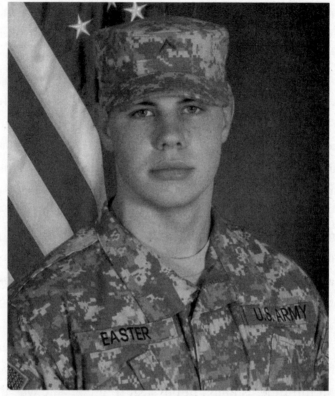

*Zac had always wanted to be an "Army badass,"
so he joined the Iowa Army National Guard.*

beating Miller by sixty-some points. In 2013, Zac was chosen from
the company to represent it at a state-level competition for the First
Battalion, 133rd Infantry Regiment. The competition tested physical training, shooting skills, and military knowledge. Zac won the
competition and was named soldier of the year for the entire Iowa
National Guard.

Superiors pointed to him as a model soldier. He twice won the
Commanders Coin of Excellence, and he earned his airborne wings.
"He was a truly bright young man who chose to be in the infantry

because he wanted to do what the infantry does," said Father Jacob Greiner, the chaplain for Zac's battalion. "He thought he could do the most good by being one of the guys who kicked down doors. With Zac everything was a challenge. He saw a challenge and wanted to beat that. Everyone who knew Zac Easter said he was one of the best." He was respected so much that he was named his company's guidon bearer, meaning that in formations he had carried the flag that represented the unit. That was a big honor. First Lt. Chase Wells, Zac's platoon leader, regarded him as someone a football coach would call a good locker room guy: Someone who was smiling and laughing, confident but never a jerk, smart enough to do things higher than his rank but committed to being part of his team.

After Zac participated in the US Army Air Assault School—a ten-day course designed to prepare soldiers for things like rappelling out of transportation and assault helicopters on insertion or evacuation missions—commanders approached him about becoming part of the 75th Ranger Regiment, an elite airborne light infantry unit in the army. Zac was stunned, and thrilled. It was a dream, to become a US Army Ranger, among the biggest badasses in a military filled with badasses: His vision of the ideal man. They gave him a packet and sent him home to think about the possibility. When Zac told his father, Myles was immediately worried. The wars in Afghanistan and Iraq would mean certain danger for someone like an Army Ranger. The father who'd sent his son into harm's way on the football field, a place where that harm used to seem pretty innocuous, was terrified of sending his son into harm's way on the battlefield. When the military told Zac there was a backlog for Ranger school, his dad was relieved. Zac was put in a holding pattern for this Army Ranger dream. His parents urged him to enroll in more college classes while he waited.

On the surface, Zac looked like the perfect candidate to become an army badass. Below the surface, though, he was coming apart. His military buddies saw hints of it from time to time. Miller and Zac did basic training together. They were fast friends, battle buddies, each other's first partners as soldiers in training. One of the drills they did in training had to do with land navigation. Commanders gave them a protractor and told them it was their most important navigation tool. Again and again, the commanders drilled it into their brains: "DO NOT lose this protractor." Zac lost his immediately. He had no idea where it went. The commanders were furious.

The biggest reason Zac wasn't quite the soldier his superiors thought he could become was because of something he kept secret. When he filled out his military medical forms, he lied about his history of concussions in football. But the concussions would continue to come. Zac wrote: "I still felt all the post concussion symptoms during basic [training, at Fort Benning] and I remember having an m-4 [a type of military assault rifle] fall on my head one time when I was sleeping because my buddy accidently knocked it over. I finished the last two weeks of basic with pounding headaches and was scared to say anything because I was scared of being recycled. With in a few weeks of getting home I got reended at a stop light by the catholic church. I was at a dead stop trying to turn and my car was totaled by a girl who hit me going like 45 mph so she says. I was instantly dazed and confused with ofcoarse a head pounding headache. The paramedics came and said I most likely had a concussion and that I should go to the hospital. Ofcouse the tough guy zac lied and told him I was fine and that im pretty sure I didn't have a concussion. I ended up going home that night."

Another time, at the beginning of a training session, the soldiers got in formations. Commanders called out their names, and they were supposed to hop out of formation when their name was called. "Easter!" a commander shouted. No answer. "Easter!" No one moved. "EASTER!" "Moving!" Zac finally replied, and he jumped out of the formation. At the time, these seemed like momentary lapses in Zac's upward trajectory. In retrospect, they seem more like clues that he was crumbling.

"I used the army to mask what I was really dealing with inside," Zac wrote, "and fed my family with all types of things about how I was going to do ROTC and go special forces when really I knew I couldn't think enough to be in ROTC and I knew that I wasn't mentally tough enough anymore for special forces. My family looked up to me so much for my military decision that I just couldn't tell them about how I felt."

So much of his energy he now devoted to making sure nobody could tell what was really going on with him. "Anything I've portrayed to anyone in the past 6 years has been a lie to conceal my secret struggle," Zac wrote. "I wish back then I knew why I was how I was and that the concussions changed me, but how was I to know when no one knew what they knew know about the repercussions of using your head as a weapon back then. I always lied to the doctors so none of them mentioned that I might eventually have a shit ton of problems."

LIFE AFTER HIGH school turned into a roller coaster of diminishing returns. The highs were never as high as Zac wanted, and the lows became ever-deepening troughs. There was one high, though—one happy, healthy, authentic high—that would stick with Zac for the rest of his life. It started on December 31, 2010, New Year's Eve. Zac was home from winter break after his first semester of college. One of Myles II's friends was having a party at his parents' house, which was out in the country, surrounded by cornfields. Zac decided to go. There was beer pong. Music blared. Zac was drunk. No, Zac was *hammered*.

Walking down a hallway, red Solo cup in hand, he saw an old friend: Alison Epperson, tall, buxom, and beautiful, a whip-smart cheerleader with a sharp wit. They'd always hit it off in high school as a yin and a yang: Zac as the good-ole-boy conservative who loved guns, football, and the military, and Ali as a feisty young woman who didn't shy away from political arguments as a liberal in this rural sea of Republicans. She was a tomboy, a lifelong fan of the Baltimore Orioles, a spitfire with striking red lips and a flirtatious smile. She loved to party, but she was more responsible about it than Zac, perhaps the lingering effect of her best friend in middle school being killed by a drunk driver. Ali was a year behind Zac in school, and the two had been friends for a couple of years. She used to skip her fourth-period music class to hang with Zac and his friend Jake in the hallways. From the start, there was a spark between the two, even if they ignored it at first. They would go to Subway and get breakfast sandwiches, then they would eat them on the senior bench.

On this New Year's Eve, exactly twenty-eight years from the night when Zac's mother and father shared their first kiss, Ali wobbled up to Zac in the hallway. She had a Monster Energy drink laced with vodka in hand. It was her eighteenth birthday, and she was tying one on. She and Zac talked and laughed. Slyly, they brushed arms. For a moment, they were alone in a corner of the house, and Zac grabbed Ali's hand and tugged her toward the door. One of Myles II's friends gave them a knowing look as they walked into the winter air.

The temperature was about to dip into the single digits: "Cold as shit, so cold," Ali recalled. They stopped by a car and shared their

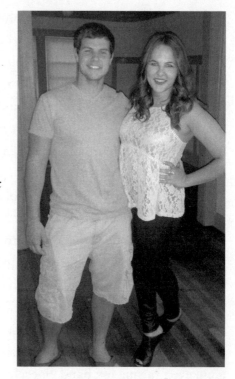

On New Year's Eve 2010, Zac and Ali shared their first kiss.

first kiss. "Oh, wow," Zac said. "This is a long time coming." They crept into an old wooden hay barn. The space was dark. Against a bale of hay, they kissed, and kissed some more. Their clothes fell to the floor. Goosebumps rose all over both of them. They rolled to the dusty ground, and they made love. "For me, from that moment on, it was always Zac—my heart was always Zac's," Ali said. They put their clothes back on and they laughed. Then, they crept back into the party, both drunkenly thinking they'd pulled off something sneaky, something that no one else would ever know about.

But it turned out that everybody already knew. *Of course* everybody knew: Their clothes were covered with straw.

    *   *   *

"I WANTED TO prove to myself that I'm not actually stupid and that I'm still the old Zac Easter who can push through anything," Zac wrote. He was writing about his early twenties, a time in his life when he dropped out of Kirkwood Community College, moved back in with his parents, and enrolled at a community college nearby. "I started off living at home for a year and a half and hardly talked to anyone. I felt so insecure with my self-image and I often never could get myself to ever talk to anyone in classes [at Des Moines Area Community College] or even talk in a class in general. I think this is when I first started panic/anxiety attacks. It seemed like anyone I tried to talk to someone other than my family I would start to panic, start sweating, get a [blushy] face, and have an insanely high heart rate. Speech classes were the worst. 10 minutes before I even got up to speak I would be soaked in sweat just sitting there . . . I worked hours on end for good grades but often didn't speak to anyone in my classes and my anxiety stopped me from even raising my hand. Speech class was the worst. I remember feeling so embarrassed and blushy faced trying to fumble through a speech."

After spending his freshman year at Kirkwood, Zac had returned to his childhood bedroom. He often felt like a failure, but he'd will himself to rally back to those roller-coaster peaks. He signed up for classes at the second community college with a vague idea of eventually going to business school. He got down on himself for feeling dumb in his classes, read a Tony Robbins self-help book for motivation, then got pumped up and scribbled down all his life goals. He got a job as a server at a Red Robin burger joint near the giant mall in Des Moines's western suburbs to prove to himself that he could be good when communicating with people. But he experienced terrifying struggles just talking with customers.

He forgot their orders, he got annoyed by their demands, and he quit the job. He lost all motivation to become an Army Ranger because he presumed he was too mentally weak—and he drank by himself and got depressed. He read Stephen R. Covey's *The 7 Habits of Highly Effective People: Powerful Lessons in How People Change*. And while he was still taking classes, he also worked for his dad, who had found himself a good gig at a mortgage company in Indianola. Then, Zac quit that job. Up, then down. Down, then up. He couldn't find a steady trajectory.

He moved to the family's farmhouse near the timber to establish independence from his parents. One lonely night, depressed, he even loaded up the .22-caliber rifle before again talking himself out of suicide. He worked out on an insane schedule: a six-mile run every morning and an intense CrossFit session every night because working out was the only thing that could help his head feel right. He struggled with sleep and became addicted to sleeping pills. After getting an associate's degree from community college, he transferred to the same four-year university in Des Moines his older brother had graduated from, Grand View University, determined to do right. He didn't make friends in classes, partly because he was too anxious, partly because he told himself he was there to get a college degree, not just to mess around like he had in Iowa City. He worked his tail off for classes and held down various jobs as he moved toward graduation. He needed to prove to himself he could make it.

No question, Zac had weathered ups and downs since high school. But, his parents thought, he was finally on track. From the outside looking in, his life seemed mostly good. That was by design. Zac's whole persona—the concussions, the military, the tough-it-out Easter mentality—had made him skilled at masking his feelings.

But a mother knows. And as Zac progressed through college, Brenda could sense things weren't right with her middle son. After Zac moved out of his parents' house and to the farmhouse, Brenda knew there was one surefire way she could bring Zac (and his brothers) back home: food. Every Sunday, she'd fix a big lunch for the family. Some weeks, it was roast beef, mashed potatoes, and vegetables. Other weeks, it was steaks with potato casserole and green beans. She'd make triple batches and send the boys home with plenty of food to get them through the week.

Brenda and Zac had always been close. When he was living at home, they'd do errands together. When Brenda was cooking on these Sundays, he'd sit in the kitchen and chat with her. As Zac roller-coastered through his postadolescence, Brenda noticed his life subtly but consistently taking on a darker tinge.

"He'd come home, and you could see he was troubled but didn't want to talk about it," Brenda later recalled to me. "Even to this day, my mother, the minute she sees me, she can tell if I'm sick, if I'm off. Mothers just can sense things about their kids. And I could see it in his eyes. I'd ask him, 'What's going on? What's new?' He was always quiet about it. But I saw distance in his eyes."

COLLEGE WAS NEARLY over. Somehow, against all odds, Zac was about to get his degree. His older brother helped him get a job working alongside him at a full-service financial firm in Des Moines's suburbs. Working with Myles II, Zac thought, was at least supposed to be exciting, and it would maybe give him a bit of that brothers-in-arms feeling he used to have on the football field. The two decided they were going to get rich, and quick. At the beginning of each workday, the brothers would pound on their chests like Matthew McConaughey's character in *The Wolf of Wall*

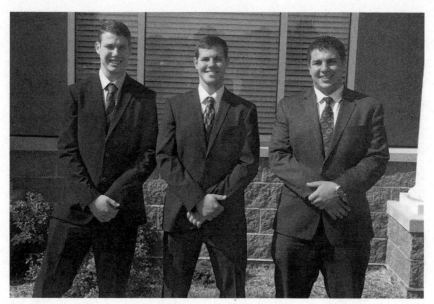

The Easter boys, (from left) Levi, Zac, Myles II.

Street: "Let's go to WORK!" At the end of the days, his brother would ask Zac if he'd made any sales. Usually, the answer was no. Zac spoke about going to business school, about investing in the stock market, about becoming a millionaire and purchasing a really nice car to replace Old Red, his 2008 cherry-red Mazda3.

It was all a ruse. In truth, Zac was coming apart. Yeah, he was working out, but part of that was to mask an addiction to fast food that he often couldn't control. Forget succeeding at work; most days, it was a struggle even to show up. Part of his job was to make cold calls to potential clients, trying to sell them insurance. But his memory was failing him, and often his language was, too. So Zac had to write a two-page script that he would follow, word for word, during sales calls. His colleagues noticed. They thought it was weird he couldn't just wing it for a standard phone call. Even with the script, he sometimes couldn't make it through a call. He'd be talking, and then all of a sudden, no words would come. Just frozen. Zac called these moments brain tremors. It felt like when a muscle in your leg cramps up—but for Zac, the cramping muscle was the brain. Sometimes, he'd have a brain tremor when he was driving, and he would have to pull over until his mind calmed down. A tremor would last up to five seconds, brief but intense pains in his head that rendered him motionless. He wondered what was going on: *Maybe a brain tumor?*

"I'm still not sure what to do about work," Zac wrote in his journal. "Right now I feel unmotivated towards it and I would like to get my shit figured out. It's also depressing knowing I have memory issues and language issues when I work in sales. All my hard work probably won't pay off . . . I didn't have any fast food binges today but I thought about it when I woke up. I feel like my body temp might be a little off because I'm sweating all the time. Jake invited me to go out to Buffalo Wild Wings with some friends. Just thinking about it gave me extreme anxiety and I felt very avoidant right away. When is this going to stop? 24 years old and I feel like I need to be hidden. I used the excuse I'm not feeling well. I was doing some research on TBI's [traumatic brain injuries] and found something about impulsive sexual behavior. Explains why all I want to do is jerk off."

Zac obsessed over his failures at work. With Tony Robbins's books at his side—one was titled *Awaken the Giant Within: How to Take Immediate Control of Your Mental, Emotional, Physical & Financial Destiny!*—Zac scrawled action plans for his success in one of his journals. "I have so much potential," Zac wrote. "If get better at cold calling and get better w/ people, I will have total self confidence and nothing will stop me. Change mentality first.

Action determines results." It's as if Zac was acting as his own therapist, his own life coach. "I just know I'll be rich and I will do it. I can overcome my fear. Practicing certainty in the mind is the most powerful thing." On one side of a sheet of paper, he scribbled empowering beliefs. ("I always outwork ppl." "I have a sexy body." "I am an athlete." "I will be a CEO.") On the other side, he scribbled disempowering beliefs. ("I'm chubby." "I'm socially awkward.") "Stop using words that disempower you and use words that empower you!" Zac wrote. "I have come far as fuck in life, and I don't even realize it."

He laid out a set of life goals. Some seemed charmingly simple; others seemed impossibly out of reach:

3 months – get stronger, 6 pack

2 months – get over red face and fear of judgement

3 months – learn stocks

1 month – get your connection w/ God back

1 month – quit chew and Adderall

1 year – get MBA

1 year – get investment certificate

2 year – become portfolio manager

1 week – post more on social media

Get into good MBA program, make 100K, drive sexy car

5 year – want to be a millionaire by age 28

1 month – want to stop spending money on stuff I don't need

2 year – motorcycle

2 year – travel USA

10 year – see a foreign country

5 year – Super Bowl

1 year – more Packers games

Zac's moods ping-ponged between an unrealistic sort of con-
quer-the-world optimism and complete hopelessness. Around the
time he was graduating from Grand View University in the spring
of 2015, Zac went to a local doctor to discuss his depression. He
asked whether he should start taking antidepressants. The doctor
gave him a pep talk. He told Zac he was a great guy, told him his
own daughter thought Zac was the greatest guy ever, told him he
needed to pray more. Then, he prescribed Zac a low-dose antidepressant. Zac asked if all his concussions could have played a part
in his depression. No, the doctor told Zac. Concussions don't do
that to somebody. Zac took the antidepressants for a month. But
he felt worse, and more depressed.

"I was determined I would make it and succeed and guess what,
nothing ended up working," Zac wrote. "I started drinking and
getting so shitfaced I often started pissing the bed and started to
have my drinking problem come back. Some nights I would tell
my friends and roommate I'm busy and sit in my room and drink
alone. Before my senior year [in college] I also got a prescription of
Adderall because I thought I had adhd. All I did was start abusing
the Adderall right away. When I picked up my first prescription
I went home and snorted several lines. The Adderall binges and
drinking binges took its toll on me. . . . It seemed the only [way]
I could get myself to seem smart and outgoing was to be high on
amphetamines from the Adderall."

The situation didn't improve. "I kept going out on the weekends
and drinking my ass off though and using any drug I could find,"
Zac wrote. "I still feel guilty because I feel like I let my brother
down by saying how I was going to be the next wolf of wall street,
but in reality, I struggled like a motherfucker to even show up. I
hid all this from everyone I knew of course and still didn't know

how to open up to people to tell them how I felt. The summer was rough at work and rough at home . . . I love my family to death, but I felt like I was snapping on them for no reason some days and I could see that somethings I said were hurting them. It just seemed like anything and everything would want to set me off."

Things weren't going any better with Zac and his friends. "Socially I was even more fucked up. I felt extremely insecure with myself and literally couldn't talk to anyone cus of my anxiety. I felt like I couldn't connect with anyone because my emotions were so fucked and I felt like I needed to stay in my room."

Without his family knowing—telling Ali but no one else—Zac started going to someone for help. Her name was Kamela Kleppe-Yeager, and her office was near the state capitol building in Des Moines. She was a speech-language pathologist, specializing in patients with concussions. In their first meeting, they talked about his issues. He brought up the concussions. She changed the wording for him, having him call the concussions "minor brain injuries." That sort of wording helped Zac process what his brain had suffered through. This wasn't just getting his bell rung on the football field; this was potentially something much more serious. She gave Zac a screening test that assessed five areas of function: his attention, his memory, his language processing, his problem solving, and his visual and spatial skills. His testing showed problems with memory and language, affirming issues Zac thought were affecting his everyday life. She noticed a delay in his speaking patterns. His brain only appeared to be able to retain memory for only about three minutes. "You sort of got a deer-in-the-headlights feeling—I saw that on Zac's face a lot," Kleppe-Yeager later recalled. "That level of internal frustration. And that interferes with your ability to problem-solve because you really freeze up. Tears would get in his eyes, but he wouldn't actually cry. He'd become more quiet. What I wanted him to do was say it, talk out loud. And he would just freeze up."

Zac kept going back to her once or twice a week, fourteen times in all over the course of a few months in the spring and summer of 2015, as he was finishing college. She taught him how to develop a "working memory," sharing simple techniques for retaining information. Taking copious notes. Setting multiple calendar reminders. Breaking up life problems into manageable chunks instead of looking at them as huge and chaotic. A healthy brain does that normally. A brain that's not healthy—Zac's brain—has to work hard to make sense of things like that. Instead of letting the information fall apart in his brain, Kleppe-Yeager taught Zac how to stitch pieces together. At one appointment, she gave him a worksheet filled with numbers and words. After a few minutes working on it, Zac started to get stressed. He had difficulty even reading the words. He felt nauseous. He told her he was having a panic attack. She said that's what they were trying to fix. She asked Zac what he did for fun, and he couldn't answer. Nothing seemed fun anymore. He told her he was always confused, and that he didn't know himself anymore. She told him he needed to take antidepressants and see a neurologist.

Zac scheduled more visits with Kleppe-Yeager, but one, two, three times, he just didn't show up. Kleppe-Yeager could only guess why Zac stopped coming. He'd made steps in the right direction, but he had a long way to go. "It was like Zac knew what he wanted to say, but he couldn't say it," Kleppe-Yeager later lamented to me. "Some people do a better job of coping. Zac didn't get that far."

After only four months, he quit the job working with his brother.

* * *

WITH HIS MEMORY failing him, Zac figured writing things down in a journal could only help. At times, the journal seemed like his best friend—the only one other than Ali he could open up to. One night in the spring of 2015, he pulled out a pen and at 9:40 p.m. started scrawling on the lined pages of a black spiral-bound Five Star Mead notebook.

"I guess today really wasn't that bad," Zac wrote. "Instead of taking the antidepressant I went and refilled my Adderall script. Popped two 30 mgs and I felt like I was at least able to get myself to do something productive. Still had the mood swings throughout the day but at least got a nice euphoric feeling listening to music, cleaning, and playing Clash of Clans all day. My dad actually called me today and wanted to chat . . . I went for a 20 min jog today, just like usual, I got dizzy and walked about every other minute. I went like 1.4 miles in 20 mins. Pretty sad since I used to do like 4-8 miles at a 7 minute pace give or take . . . that makes me depressed . . . I feel like I've gained 10-15 pounds uncontrollably. The impulse binging needs to stop, but I don't know how when I don't even know I'm doing it.

"Even with two 30 mg Adderall in me and about another 10 mgs I poored out and snorted, I still got lost all around Menards and the Dollar Store . . . IDK what it was but I felt like I kept walking all around the store and passed what I was looking for several times. I straight up felt confused on what I was looking and kept forgetting even right after I looked at my list. I only went for like 3 things too . . . I only have about a 3 minute memory after that I'm fucked. I even took three wrong turns on the way home. Shit happens I guess."

The next day, Zac was driving to Indianola from Des Moines, a thirty-minute drive that he'd made hundreds if not thousands of times before. He was almost in a trance and nearly hit a car. He got lost on the way to his parents' house.

For hours at a time, starting that senior year of college and going into the summer after graduation, Zac would go online and research the postconcussion symptoms that he thought were wrecking his life. He wondered whether this nightmare was the price of playing football, the sport he'd loved his entire life—the sport that, let's be honest, he still loved, even if it contributed to his ruin. He kept reading about this scary-sounding degenerative disease of the brain that presented like Alzheimer's but appeared in ex-athletes from contact sports decades before Alzheimer's would typically set in. It sounded like a scientific word salad: *chronic traumatic encephalopathy*. He couldn't even spell it correctly, but the symptoms all sounded familiar: Memory problems. Personality changes. Mood swings between depression and aggression. He read about former NFL stars who'd been diagnosed with this terrifying disease, but only after they died, often by suicide. Zac watched a PBS documentary about NFL Hall of Famer Mike Webster, who was essentially Patient Zero in the developing public health crisis surrounding this brain disease among former football players.

"Some days I feel like IDK who I am anymore," Zac wrote. "I've noticed I'm relying on drugs to try and be who I want to be. I need to stop, but at the same time I'm like Fuck it . . . I wont lie, I feel kind of scared and depressed about my future. I found some info online about CTE and got scared . . . I just wish I could be my old self and understand whats going on."

His old self seemed to be a ghost, replaced by this new person he didn't particularly like. "My motivation has been slacking and I feel pretty depressed. I feel like I need to abuse Adderall to get anything done as far as talking to ppl. My impulse control seems to be getting worse. I just want to go on huge food binges and I can't stop. Also have been feeling very impatient with people and feel like I just want to snap something. I miss the old Zac."

THROUGH IT ALL, the main person he confessed these vulnerabilities to was Ali. They'd been an on-again, off-again item since that New Year's Eve they'd made love in the freezing-cold barn. She'd left Iowa for college at a private school in a small town in Kentucky. They were able to live their own lives when she was at school, each dating other people, each having plenty of wild times. But they would text nonstop and talk on the phone. When she was home from college, they were virtually inseparable.

They thought their relationship was their big secret, that their friends didn't know. They'd be at a bar in downtown Des Moines with a group of friends, and when one of them said their special code phrase—"Rum and Coke?"—they'd disappear together. They'd talk. They'd make up goofy dances on the dance floor. They'd make out. She loved how silly he was around her—she seemed to be the only person he could be like that around—and she loved what a thoughtful and thoroughly decent young man he was. For five years they played this game. "We'd always go back to each other—that was the one constant," Ali said later. They got out of their small town and went on nondate dates in the big city, just the two of them: To P.F. Chang's near the mall, to Zombie Burger + Drink Lab near the state capitol building in Des Moines's industrial East Village, to Sakari Sushi Lounge on the Ingersoll Avenue commercial strip. He called her by a pet name: "Winslow," her middle name. It was only when they were drunk when some other words would slip out: "I love you."

But at some point during the summer of 2015, something started to change. Maybe it was because Ali was going to be moving to Cleveland, Ohio, at the end of the summer to attend Case Western Reserve University School of Law, so their time together felt short. Maybe it was because Ali was the only person who Zac felt he could spill everything out to about these worsening troubles inside his brain. He swore her to secrecy on all of it; don't tell anyone, Zac instructed, but especially not his parents. But that summer, a relationship that had been casual started to become something much more. They went on long walks around Gray's Lake, an old gravel mine near an oxbow in the Raccoon River with a perfectly framed view of downtown Des Moines's skyline. They went to the beach at Lake Ahquabi near Zac's parents' house, threw clumps of grass at each other, and stared at the clouds as children and their parents rented paddleboats. They held hands, first in the dark, at a movie theater, and eventually in public. "You're the mac to my cheese," Zac texted her. She calmed him more than anyone. She convinced him that he needed to tell his family what was happening. She told him that, no matter what was going on with his brain, they would figure it out. Together.

On the night of his twenty-fourth birthday, Zac Easter and his cousin Cole Fitzharris met at the Sports Page Grill in Indianola, ordered Coors Lights, and waited for Zac's parents to arrive. Zac was nervous. His cousin could hear it in his voice. By this point, June of 2015, not quite six years since his final football game, Zac had become convinced that his five diagnosed concussions (plus who knows how many more that were never diagnosed) across a decade of using his head as a weapon had triggered his downward spiral.

Meanwhile, Zac's parents believed their son was on top of the world. Somehow, through a combination of hard work and faking it, he'd just graduated from college, and even made the honor roll his final semester. Last they heard, he was considered a star in the Iowa National Guard, maybe even bound for Army Ranger school if things broke the right way. They approved of this relationship with Ali, and they loved the fact that it was inching toward something real and special. A full life awaited their middle child.

But his parents were buying into the mirage: the degree, the girl, the job, the stability. He'd just asked his first postgraduation employer for some time off from work when his parents arrived for his birthday dinner. Zac took an anxious swig from his Coors Light, gathered himself, then told them he needed to talk.

"Something's been going on with my head," he began.

From there, he laid it all out: He was quitting his job because he needed to focus on his health. He was often tired and dizzy and nauseated. He got headaches all the time. Sometimes while driving, he'd go into these trances; he'd snap out of it when he drove his car into a curb. Panic attacks came without warning. He had started writing down a long list of questions for his doctor; one of them was "Do you think I'm showing signs of CTE or dementia?" In fact, he already knew the answer to that one. He had just visited a doctor who specialized in concussions and who told him that, yes, he very well might have CTE.

His parents were stunned. They knew some things were off. Sometimes on the phone it sounded like Zac was talking with marbles in his mouth. And they'd noticed that his bank account, which they still had access to, was suddenly hemorrhaging money. But mostly, they just assumed their son was a young man grappling with the growing pains of adulthood and independence.

Now, though, he was telling them that he might have a mysterious brain disease that afflicted NFL players, haunting them for decades after their careers had ended. One psychologist even told Zac that he would end up penniless, homeless, and in a mental institution. Not could. *Would*. Zac had walked out of that guy's office terrified.

Myles Easter Sr. had seen the news reports of ex-NFL stars whose lives unraveled postretirement and ended in suicide. Mike Webster, Andre Waters, Dave Duerson, Junior Seau, the Sunday gladiators who once were the apotheosis of all that he worshipped about the game of football. But Myles never really believed this disease existed. To be honest, even the mention of it kind of disgusted him. CTE was an excuse, he had always thought: a bunch of millionaire athletes who'd had it made, who blew through all their money, who fell out of the limelight, who got depressed, who then killed themselves. But now, hearing his own son—still just a kid, no jaded pro, someone who had never played a day of football above the high school level—say that he might have CTE?

"It just caught me so off guard," Myles Sr. said later. "I was honestly dumbfounded."

The dinner table went quiet. Then, Brenda, Zac's mom, broke the silence.

"Well," she said, "let's fix it."

SEVEN

The Doctor

THE FIRST TIME Zac Easter steered Old Red into Dr. Shawn Spooner's sports medicine clinic, in a well-manicured strip mall in suburban Des Moines, Zac couldn't have known he was about to meet a kindred spirit. Spooner has the boy-next-door look that could make older patients uncertain whether he's just some medical-school student on rotation: a buzz cut and a hint of a lisp, warm brown eyes and an easy smile, the limber muscles of an avid road cyclist, and the earnest manner of a doctor who really listens to your problems. Like Zac, Spooner grew up in small-town Iowa, in Kingsley, a speck of a town not far from where Iowa, Nebraska, and South Dakota converge, and a childhood home of US President Herbert Hoover. Like Zac, Spooner had played football in high school and still loves the sport. And like Zac at the time of his first appointment, Spooner had taken a recent interest in concussions. Zac had visited plenty of people to help his broken brain: therapists and psychiatrists, family practice doctors and neurologists. Few gave him confidence they were the right person to fix it, until Zac walked into this building one spring day in 2015.

On Zac's first visit, the doctor quizzed him on his head issues. It wasn't like Zac's speech was horribly slurred, but it didn't take long for Spooner's alarm bells to go off: Zac told him about previous concussions, in football and otherwise, and about how things were getting worse even though it had been several years since his last concussion. He told the doctor about his trouble focusing, and his up-and-down emotions, and the drinking and drugs he used to cope. The fact Zac was still struggling with what seemed like post-concussion symptoms for years after his last concussion was concerning. What had started Zac's downward spiral—whether it was the concussions or preexisting mental health issues or some toxic cocktail of both—didn't matter so much to Spooner as where Zac stood right now: isolated, anxious, socially avoidant. Zac spoke of the facade he put up even to himself; he was telling himself he was training to be an Army Ranger, but deep down, he knew that was a lie. He talked about his depression. Shortly before meeting Spooner, Zac wrote this in his journal: "Thoughts of suicide are creeping in my head and its freaking me out."

Zac seemed confused by the conflicting media reports he'd read about CTE in former football players. He didn't know which sources to trust. That confusion had morphed into fear and anxiety. *This young man,* Spooner thought, *is the exact type who can fall through the cracks and never get help.* Spooner ordered an MRI to get a detailed look at Zac's brain and brain stem to see if an image would show anything awry: a brain tumor, perhaps. From that very first appointment, it occurred to Spooner that Zac's symptoms so many years after concussions could be a case of CTE, which can't be positively diagnosed until after death, through an autopsy and studying the brain.

But Spooner was cautious of drawing a simple straight line from concussions to postconcussion syndrome to chronic neurological impairment to CTE. Science takes time to come to a consensus. There was far from a scientific consensus on how concussions and subconcussive events affect the human brain, whose system of one hundred billion connected neurons has been called "the most complicated object in the known universe." Any conclusion Spooner could come to about what Zac was experiencing inside his skull, and why he was experiencing it, was nothing more than a very educated guess. Maybe this young man really was experiencing an incredibly early onset of CTE. Or maybe it was something else. Most likely, Spooner thought, it was a nasty stew of many things: Zac's brain struggling to recover from years of punishing football hits, but also his mental health and substance abuse issues, which may or may not be related to concussions. Science and medicine are messy and inexact, more art than math. What Spooner discerned from the five years since high school ended for Zac was that this sounded like a bad reaction to multiple concussions that were never properly treated. And this was the type of thing Spooner had become intimately acquainted with in the same period of time as Zac's descent.

Zac's childhood had been remarkably similar to his new doctor's. Spooner's dad ran a John Deere dealership in their town of fifteen hundred people, where his mom was a dental hygienist. In high school, Spooner did it all: He ran track, acted in the school play, and played plenty of sports, from football to basketball to baseball. He was a voracious reader. It was a big moment when *Sports Illustrated* and *National Geographic* arrived on the same day. He worked his way up to the scientific treatises of Stephen Hawking. Football was his favorite sport. Just to field an eleven-man team in their district, players had to play both sides of the ball, so Spooner, all five-foot-eleven and 175 pounds of him, played center and nose tackle. The team was horrible. It didn't matter; the games and even the practices were among the greatest times of Spooner's life. "It's just the cumulative experience of being on a team, with the guys," Spooner told me. "Whatever, we weren't good. But the experience wouldn't have been any different."

He went to Iowa State University to become a physical trainer. His first two years he spent his time in the athletic training room, taping up Cyclone football players, setting up the whirlpool for basketball players, working the ultrasound machine to treat pain for wrestlers. But physical training was too static and monotonous for Spooner; he wanted to be where the action was, and the action seemed to be with the doctors. So he applied to University of Iowa's Carver College of Medicine in Iowa City. "I grew up in a small town, and all we had was a family doctor," Spooner said. "He did everything—casts, delivered babies, anything. This was what I wanted to be, the guy you go to when you need something."

But medical school is expensive. Something caught Spooner's eye as he was looking through his acceptance paperwork: the Health Professions Scholarship Program. It was the summer of 2001, the end of a golden, conflict-free time in the US military. The United States hadn't been in a conflict lasting more than six months since Vietnam. In exchange for free schooling, he committed to mandatory military service. Spooner picked the navy; his dad and his cousins had served in the navy, so why not? He attended the navy's officer indoctrination course in Newport, Rhode Island, basically five weeks during which medical-school students learned to salute and to wear their navy uniform right, then reported to Iowa City for medical school. He spent one summer in a hospital in Boone, Iowa, living in an unused patient room, hanging out in the emergency room, and going on ambulance runs. When he graduated, a naval officer met him on the lawn outside the U of I's Hancher Auditorium and promoted him to lieutenant. Along with his new bride, he reported to Camp Pendleton between Los Angeles and San Diego, one of the largest Marine Corps bases in the country, to complete his family medicine residency.

During his second year, he was stationed on the obstetrics floor, delivering scores of babies. Late one night, a doctor he was working with mentioned he was part of the base's sports fellowship program. Spooner spent the rest of the evening quizzing the doctor on the program, which seemed to marry Spooner's two great interests: sports and medicine. After being deployed to South Korea for two years, where his second child was born, he returned to San Diego for the one-year sports medicine fellowship, then was sent to the Naval Station Great Lakes near Chicago, where he worked in the sports medicine clinic.

One weekend in the fall of 2012, a few months before his required military service was up, Spooner, his wife, and their three children—the youngest had been born just weeks before—were visiting family in Iowa. They were going through a corn maze near Spooner's parents' home when his cell phone rang. It was his naval commander. His commander knew Spooner had only a short time left in his commitment, which meant he wasn't eligible for a long overseas deployment. But the commander also knew there were only a couple of dozen sports medicine doctors in the navy, and one was needed in Afghanistan. The commander was to the point: "You're up," he said. "You don't have to go. We'll fight it for you. But it would be great if you went."

The military had paid for his schooling, and Spooner had served his required time. But he hadn't really done anything operational. "It's like being on a football team and standing on the sidelines," Spooner said. "I wanted to be part of it. I felt like it was my obligation." In a way, this was Spooner's test of manhood. He looked at his wife, who held their new baby. It wasn't a long conversation. "Yep, I'll do it," he told his commander. He had twenty-eight days before his departure. The next day, a real estate agent showed them five houses in Des Moines's suburbs, and they put in a full-price offer for one. One box checked off before his nine-month deployment.

Spooner went through predeployment training, brushing up on his firearms skills and learning how to burst into a house and clear a room. Then, on a dreary day in January 2013, he sat in a big, gray, windowless Boeing C-17 Globemaster III military transport plane alongside two hundred other military members. The flight from the staging area in Kyrgyzstan to the war zone in Afghanistan was somber. The landing was steep to avoid potential rocket attacks; it felt like the plane might crash. He arrived at Camp Leatherneck, the huge base in southern Afghanistan's Helmand Province, the single deadliest province for the coalition troops since 2001. The doctor was at war.

The military had been dealing with the effects of concussions on servicemen since World War I, when trench warfare introduced frequent use of high explosives and artillery fire, causing head injuries. Some World War I servicemen were diagnosed with shell shock, a catch-all term that encapsulated problems with memory and sleeping, and with headaches and depression. The scientific community at the time was divided, much like it is today, about whether physical injury was the primary cause of these symptoms, or whether they had more to do with preexisting mental health issues. Even then, the issue was clouded by politics. "Despite the lack of any pathological studies on the brains of individuals diagnosed with shell shock," Ann McKee, one of today's preeminent researchers into neurodegenerative disease, wrote with a coauthor in a 2014 paper, "wartime committees entreated with the responsibility to inquire into the entity declared the disorder to have psychiatric origins." During the Persian Gulf War in the early 1990s, the word *concussion* was hardly uttered, but by the first few years of the Iraq War about a dozen years later, concussions and traumatic brain injuries skyrocketed because of insurgents using improvised explosive devices (IEDs). At first the treatment was, essentially, here's some ibuprofen, get back to work. But as wartime concussions ramped up, and as the fledgling science indicated these were brain injuries and not just someone getting his bell rung, the military started taking them more seriously.

Not coincidentally, this occurred simultaneously with scientists like Omalu and McKee discovering that the long-term problems associated with concussions were far greater than originally thought. Two studies in 2009 and 2010 indicated that the prevalence of minor traumatic brain injuries—concussions—among returning service members was between 15.2 percent and 22.8 percent. Concussion was the most common battlefield injury, affecting more than three hundred thousand service members since 9/11. Once leaders realized the importance of taking brain injuries seriously, the military began medevacking concussed soldiers home for recovery, which not only left personnel vacancies but also cost the government money. So in 2011, the navy opened the Concussion Restoration Care Center at Camp Leatherneck. It was the first multidisciplinary concussion rehabilitation clinic in a war zone, treating soldiers during the acute phase immediately after a concussion. This was the center Spooner was selected to lead.

The center's concept was simple and revolutionary. Because the brain is such a complex organ, it means injuries are best treated by a team of medical personnel with different specialties. Spooner's

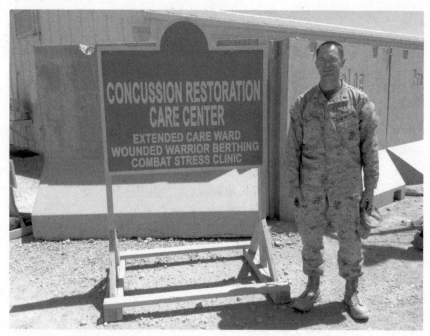

*Dr. Shawn Spooner led the Concussion Restoration Care Center
in Afghanistan's Helmand Province in 2013.*

center did neurocognitive testing on each service member to establish a baseline before the deployment. In the event of a potential concussion, injured soldiers would be kept for observation for at least forty-eight hours. Spooner was the lead physician, the quarterback of the medical team, which also included a neuropsychologist, who worked on cognition, mental recovery, and stress and anxiety management; a psychiatrist, who managed medications; a physical therapist, who dealt with musculoskeletal issues like back, neck, and shoulder injuries; and an occupational therapist, who worked on balance, functional vision, and cognitive rehabilitation.

Having all these specialists under one roof to treat concussion, a first for the military, worked. Between 2011 and the end of 2013, the Concussion Restoration Care Center treated about two thousand service members experiencing acute symptoms of concussion. Roughly 98 percent recovered within ten days and were sent back to their units. This was a huge positive for the military, and service members appreciated it as well. The sense of duty for an injured soldier who wants to return to his comrades is analogous to an injured football player eager to get back to his team: Both just want back on the playing field. At the Afghanistan concussion center, only thirty-two out of the two thousand people treated were sent home. The rest stayed on the battlefield. The most significant common factor of those thirty-two was that they had a preexisting mental health diagnosis before they were deployed and before they had a concussion. To Spooner, it appeared there was a correlation between existing mental health issues and taking longer to recover from concussion. Perhaps the link is something in the DNA, perhaps it's situational, but certain people seemed more susceptible to major struggles after a concussion.

Spooner noticed concussion recovery came in three buckets. The most obvious was physiological recovery—musculoskeletal problems, including neck and shoulder stiffness, headaches, sensitivity to light, alongside issues of balance and how you focus your vision. For doctors, this is easy to diagnose. A more difficult bucket to grasp is the metabolic recovery: How is brain chemistry changed by concussion or repeated subconcussive events? There's research being done on animal brains to study what happens to a brain in the acute stage of a concussion. But it's not like scientists can cut open a human brain and study it in the days after a concussion. "That's something we just don't know yet," Spooner said. "If you really test people [who've been concussed] way past the time you'd assume they are ready to go back and play, you still have metabolic carryover that lasts longer than we thought it does. Does that mean they're more vulnerable to head injuries later? We don't know yet."

And then there's the bucket of mental and psychosomatic recovery. The most severe postconcussion cases that Spooner has seen, the ones that last not weeks but months or years, have heavy undertones of depression and anxiety. Essentially, the concussion affects not just the patient's brain but his or her mind. An innocuous trigger can make someone dizzy or nauseous or fall to the ground. For example, someone at a grocery store encounters a person pushing a fast grocery cart in his or her direction and flips out. The emotional response could be an expression of preexisting mental health issues made worse by the concussion; it could be a manifestation of post-traumatic stress disorder. For a doctor, the diagnosis is often guesswork.

What Spooner doesn't want is for hysteria to develop over football and concussions—a presumption that multiple concussions always lead to depression, then anxiety, then suicide, then an autopsy that diagnoses CTE. "Maybe they had protein tangles in their brain. Or maybe not. When I see people recover, I see them *recover*. Way more than 90 percent are better in a short period. But every concussion I see is different. It's like snowflakes. They're similar, they have similar features, but each one is different."

Just about every day during Spooner's seven months in Afghanistan, his team would get new patients. Usually, it would be a group of soldiers whose armored fighting vehicle hit an IED. They'd undergo the same concussion screening in the field that football players receive on the sideline. If they tested positive, they'd come to Spooner's center. One kid—a quiet teenage marine, straight out of high school and into the war zone—had recently arrived in Afghanistan when his vehicle ran into an IED. One of his buddies was hurt badly enough that he was sent home. The teenage marine had a concussion so severe that it took him two or three weeks at Spooner's center to recover. Then, they discharged him, and he went back to his unit.

A week later, the marine was on an isolated base staffed with soldiers from the country of Georgia; American troops were working closely with them. A suicide bomber drove a truck packed with explosives through the outer perimeter of the compound and blew himself up. The young marine was standing next to a helium tank, which exploded. That meant he was hit by the first blast wave from the original explosion and then, immediately after that, a second blast wave from the helium tank. The attack, which the Taliban took responsibility for, wiped out half the base. Seven Georgian soldiers died. The young marine was at the epicenter of mass trauma; that night, thirty-five Georgians and Americans were admitted to the one-room clinic with low lighting. It felt like *M*A*S*H*. Some had soft-tissue damage from shrapnel, but most were affected by the blasts' shock wave.

It was the most hectic night of Spooner's deployment. Staffers brought out Sharpies and wrote results of concussion evaluations on injured soldiers' forearms. Spooner can remember the look on the teenage marine's face: A week after recovering from his first concussion, he'd gotten blown up two more times in a manner of moments. His eyes looked drunk: They were foggy, staring into space. His movements were slow. So was his cognition. "He just looked sad," Spooner said. "It was more than just a concussion. It was like, *What the hell is happening to me?*" He stayed at the concussion center a while. Weeks passed. Service members were released when they showed improvement. But the marine wasn't recovering at all. He was one of those thirty-two service members who got sent home.

That marine stuck in Spooner's mind. Where did his life go from there? Would he find himself in a VA hospital years or decades later still dealing with the aftereffects of this one June night in Afghanistan? When Spooner's deployment ended and he returned to civilian life in central Iowa, he pledged to make treating concussions a central part of his sports medicine practice. Like he did in Afghanistan, Spooner constructed a program that put all the needed resources to treat complex concussions on the same team. We too often think of medicine as the newest machines and latest pharmaceuticals. But oftentimes, the best medicine is about processes. For Spooner, it was a matter of concussion patients immediately having access to neuropsychologists, physical therapists, psychiatrists, and occupational therapists, not waiting weeks or months for proper treatment.

Or, in Zac Easter's case, years.

When Zac walked into Spooner's office six years after his final football concussion and said he was still experiencing aftereffects, Spooner thought of that young marine. He saw in Zac that same deer-in-headlights look. The loss of hope. The sense that something had been permanently altered inside his brain.

So Spooner tried to give him hope.

"I felt even more paranoid with what other people thought of me and sometimes I wasn't sure if I was hearing stuff or not," Zac wrote around this time. "I know I started to become psychotic some nights here recently because I feel like I've started to become delusional or I've been kind of hearing and seeing things. A few times I've gone down stairs and have asked the guys what they wanted because I sware I heard someone calling my name. A lot of this

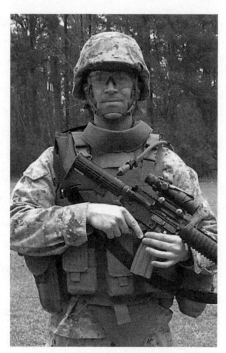

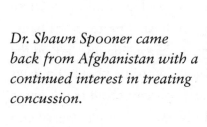

*Dr. Shawn Spooner came
back from Afghanistan with a
continued interest in treating
concussion.*

freaked me out because I'm not sure if I was going schitzo or not. I've felt like some days I've just been out of it. Over the years I've been starting to forget peoples names and just forget daily things. My roommates even joked about an alzhiemers commercial about an old lady losing her shit because I've felt like I've lost mine slowly."

Spooner had to get Zac out of his "I'm broken" funk. "You're broken," Spooner told him, "but you're not broken forever." Spooner told Zac that he shouldn't *hope* for recovery; he should *expect* recovery. Sure, he would struggle at times, like anyone with a chronic illness. But trust that you will improve, he told Zac.

On June 16, 2015, around the time of Zac's second appointment with Spooner, he scrawled an entry in his journal. His words hinted at optimism.

"My 5 year class reunion is next month and I hope I at least got my shit together by then, so I can be social, plus I don't really have any other friends," Zac wrote. "I've been to 3 colleges and always felt to scared to be close friends with someone and for some reason I could never open up to anyone. Even when I would CrossFit, it was hard for me to become 'close' friends with someone. I feel like I try to avoid any situation to go out and meet new ppl. Often times when I'm running or listening to music I pretend I'm living a different life and it keeps me going. I always imagine having the girl I was to shy to talk to and hanging with the people I always wanted to. I've always been super self conscious and try to avoid public situations when my pic could be taken. I don't even like to look at myself whether I look ripped or fat. O well—enough of the pitty party. I'm going to try and go for a run, maybe hopefully get my old self back!"

DEPENDING ON YOUR point of view, the setting for the Fifth Matthew Gfeller Sport-Related Neurotrauma Symposium was either incredibly tone-deaf—showing just how deeply in bed the football-industrial complex is with the medical and scientific communities studying brain injuries—or the only appropriate venue. I chose to see it as the latter. A couple of hundred brain scientists, athletic trainers, and other specialists, all of whom possessed knowledge of how contact sports affect the brain that far outpaced my own, strode into the third floor of Kenan Memorial Stadium at the University of North Carolina at Chapel Hill on a drizzly morning in March 2019. The college town had a special buzz because the next day North Carolina was scheduled to battle its Tobacco Road archrival, Duke, in basketball. The conference's namesake, Matthew Gfeller, had been a do-it-all boy growing up in Winston-Salem, North Carolina, as comfortable singing onstage as he was lifting in the weight room as he pursued his goal of starting as a sophomore for his high school's varsity football team. In August 2008, months after he'd become an Eagle Scout, Matthew was playing his first varsity game when he suffered a helmet-to-helmet collision. He died two days later. His parents lobbied for better concussion protocol for student-athletes and started this center to spur on concussion research.

The day I walked into the symposium, a few things stood out: That the windows looked out on the yellow goalposts, where more than fifty thousand fans convened to watch the very sport at the forefront of the concussion crisis. That the symposium was sponsored by Riddell, the helmet maker that's been sued by former NFL players with long-term health issues but every year introduces new helmets aiming to reduce concussions. That the previous football coach at UNC, Larry Fedora, had less than a year before created a firestorm by questioning the links between football and CTE, saying this: "I fear that the game will get pushed so far to one extreme you won't recognize the game 10 years from now . . . I do believe if it gets to that point that our country goes down, too." And that the keynote speaker, Dr. Allen Sills, the NFL's chief medical officer, began his presentation, titled "Is there a future for football?" with a photograph of him with NFL Commissioner Roger Goodell.

There are some who would stop right at Sills's potential conflict-of-interest disclosure—that he is a full-time paid employee of the NFL—and dismiss this conference right off the bat. Science must be independent, these people say, and cannot be subject to pressures of moneyed interests. When I told Kimberly Archie, a California attorney and one of the foremost advocates for the rights of young athletes specifically relating to concussions in football, that I was attending this conference, she bristled. (Archie lost her son, posthumously found to have CTE, in a motorcycle accident.) These North Carolina researchers have taken millions of dollars in funding from the NFL, including a three-year, $2.6 million grant announced in 2017 to study postconcussion rehabilitation techniques, therefore they were dirty. She saved a special amount of disgust for Kevin Guskiewicz, a sports medicine researcher at the University of North Carolina at Chapel Hill who is the founding director of the Matthew Gfeller Sport-Related Traumatic Brain Injury Research Center. In 2018, Guskiewicz had served as an expert witness for the defense in a lawsuit from a former University of Texas football player whose widow sought to hold the NCAA responsible for his health problems decades after his playing career ended. "He is the devil," Archie had told me about Guskiewicz. "The one place you can't play both sides of the ball is in litigation. You're either the plaintiff or the defense." Archie and others like her believe researchers who take the NFL's money are dirtied by it and cannot be trusted. Emblematic of modern-day America, even the science is politicized.

I chose to take a different view, maybe because the different view—that these researchers, scientists, and doctors are working in good faith with an NFL that's finally realized the threat of concussions—is the only view that offers hope for a solution. Sure, I would be skeptical of any broad conclusions about the future of football made by a paid employee of the NFL. But I also believe that you have to operate within the system to change the system. Guskiewicz and the Matthew Gfeller center certainly have close ties with football's power brokers. He used to work for the Pittsburgh Steelers, for example, and he's a member of the NFL's head, neck, and spine committee. But he's also an eminent scholar, a recipient of the MacArthur Fellowship "genius grant," and the chancellor at UNC. If football is to be saved, it must start at the highest level, where the most money is, and then trickle down to colleges, high schools, and youth. If that means potential conflicts of interest, well, it feels inevitable.

It's hard to imagine a more accomplished scientist to lead the NFL's efforts than Sills. He is a professor of neurological surgery at Vanderbilt University Medical Center in Nashville, and has served as a consulting neurosurgeon for Division I collegiate teams as well as NBA, NHL, and NFL franchises. He has been named eight times among America's top doctors by the Castle Connolly guide. When it comes to acknowledging concussions as a problem in football, Sills is held in much higher regard in this field of medicine than Dr. Elliot Pellman, a rheumatologist who was the New York Jets team doctor and chaired the NFL Mild Traumatic Brain Injury Committee from 1994 until 2007, or Dr. Ira Casson, who cochaired the committee from 2007 to 2009. Casson became known as Dr. No after appearing on HBO's *Real Sports* in 2007 and saying multiple head injuries caused no long-term health problems in NFL players. Together, those two became the face of the NFL's denialism of the long-term impact of football's head-jarring collisions. The NFL's head-in-the-sand period of rejecting science has been analogized to the way tobacco companies once brushed away concerns that smoking could cause cancer.

As ESPN reporters Mark Fainaru-Wada and Steve Fainaru put it in their seminal book *League of Denial: The NFL, Concussions, and the Battle for Truth*, those were "those strange years when the National Football League went to war against science." Sills is the NFL's flesh-and-blood admission that the science the league had railed against for so long was actually right. Or, as Guskiewicz stated: "CTE is real." And the existential threat to football is real, too. You don't have to look any further than the amount the NFL has invested in research—$235 million in brain injury research over the past five years, including $35 million in 2018 alone, for long-term studies about the consequences of playing football—for proof.

Sills's PowerPoint presentation about football's future first looked at the sport's past. He noted that concerns about the dangers of football are not a new problem, and he brought up those 18 football deaths and 159 serious injuries, most of them involving devastating spinal damage, in 1905. He noted the NFL has made forty-seven rule changes in the past fifteen years to improve players' health and safety. Kickoff rules in particular were dramatically changed after studies indicated those plays result in the highest number of head injuries. All players on the kickoff team now remain stationary until the ball is kicked, taking away the running start. There is now no blocking until the ball is caught, and no wedge blocks where the receiving team has two shoulder-to-shoulder blockers act as a two-person shield for the returner. The league now has thirty medical personnel at NFL stadiums on game days, including independent neurological consultants on the sidelines, support that was implemented in 2013.

NFL engineers did video analyses of every in-game concussion between 2015 and 2018 and matched each hit against 150 variables, including how the player was hurt, where the contact was initiated from, where on the helmet the contact occurred, and the force factors involved. Then, the NFL ranked all thirty-four models of helmets players are permitted to wear; helmets that fell into the green category were the best helmets, while yellow helmets were decent, and red were substandard. For the 2018 season, the NFL

Players Association banned all ten helmets from the worst tier, and about half of NFL players changed their helmet.

"No player would sign up for a shoe that has a two times greater risk of an ACL tear," Sills told the conference attendees. Ten new helmet models were introduced for 2019, he said, all in the best tier in terms of safety. The NFL's efforts seem to have made a difference. The number of in-game concussions fell 29 percent from the 2017 season to the 2018 season, from 190 concussions to 135. And there was a 27 percent reduction in all injuries on kickoff plays alone.

"Let me be very clear—we have to recognize CTE as a very real pathologic entity that's best been characterized in autopsy," Sills said. "Unfortunately, we're still somewhat in our infancy in understanding some really important factors about who gets this disease, why they get it, what are the motivating factors, are there treatment implications, and what can we possibly do to diagnose or intervene in real life. This idea that you either believe in CTE or you don't is a completely useless construct. Frankly, there is a disorder called CTE. We're all aware of that. We just need to learn more about it."

If there's one thing to take away from spending two days with a bunch of neuroscientists talking about things like how chronic pain alters brain plasticity, and how long it will take for blood-based biomarkers to move from research labs to clinical applications, it's this: how far concussion science still has to go. The phrase I heard more than any other was "the infancy of the science." Members of the media like myself want answers, and we want them fast—especially when we hear of suicides by athletic heroes like Junior Seau, who had a terrifying disease caused by the very sport we worshipped him for playing.

But the desire for immediate solutions fails to take into account how young this scientific field is. The first-ever meeting about the treatment of concussion took place in 2015. Thirty-seven international experts convened in Pittsburgh and voted on sixteen statements of agreement, later published in the journal *Neurosurgery*. These statements weren't exactly headline makers: The experts agreed concussions are treatable and characterized by diverse symptoms and impairment in function. But even these baseline agreements among scientists marked a major advancement. "If we have thirty types of knee injury, why would we think there's only one type of concussion?" asked Micky Collins, director of the Sports Medicine Concussion Program at the University of Pittsburgh Medical Center.

In recent years, the media's focus on the long-term effect of sport-related concussion as well as smaller repetitive subconcussive events has been omnipresent. Guskiewicz pointed out that the *New York Times* had published 333 articles on CTE between 2003 and 2017, yet in the world of scientific literature, there were only three hundred diagnosed cases of CTE during that same period. The media has "sort of sensationalized this at times," Guskiewicz said. "At times, though, [the media has] gotten it wrong around the later-life neurodegenerative diseases such as CTE and Alzheimer's disease, and painting this really ugly picture as if any athlete who plays contact sports for any period of time is highly likely to develop this. And that's just not the case." Science, by its very nature, is cautious. It wants to prove a hypothesis again and again before determining its value. And cautious means slow—much slower than the public, which expects a quick cure-all, can stomach. "It takes time for good research to happen," Sills said. "What can we do until we have more information?"

The good that has come out of the NFL's concussion crisis is an increased visibility of this issue, which means more money and research, which together will ideally mean a sped-up timeline. Prior to 1990, PubMed, the search engine that has more than twenty-nine million citations for biomedical literature, had a total of seven publications on sport-related concussion in its database. This research field barely existed thirty years ago. In 2018 alone, there were 216 PubMed publications on sport-related concussion. "Fifteen years ago, we really couldn't get anybody to talk about [sport-related concussion or civilian neurotrauma], and sure as hell we couldn't get anybody to fund it," said Mike McCrea, vice chair of research for the department of neurosurgery at the Medical College of Wisconsin and a leading researcher in the field. Federal funding over the past five years has surpassed $135 million. "When you think about where we started back in the late 1980s or early 1990s, believe it or not, this wasn't even recognized as quote 'injury,'" McCrea continued. "When I talked with my high school buddies, or the guys I played ball with in high school and college, it was like a subject of comic relief. It was the thing that we talked about over the summer or at our early high school reunions—'You remember when you got your head knocked off on a kick return and you were in the wrong huddle? Ha, ha!' It really had this lack of even a recognition as an injury. It was something, but not an injury."

McCrea has led research into blood-based biomarkers to diagnose concussions quickly. This is thrilling science: A biomarker is a measurable substance in the human body that can tip off scientists about diseases, infections, or, potentially, concussion. In time, the promise of blood-based biomarkers is a quick blood draw on the sideline to diagnose a concussion within minutes. But this science is, as McCrea put it, "not yet ready for prime time." Now, those blood-based biomarkers can give accurate results months later as part of a research initiative. When researchers speak about the promise of these biomarkers, the timeline is measured in decades, not years. There is, McCrea said, a "long translational bridge" between research labs and clinical applications.

But the science is real. Even as Sills was speaking at this symposium, there were four sites around the country collecting research-grade serum and plasma in potentially concussed patients and using a handheld rapid analyzer to figure out in real time if biomarkers indicated concussion. Even a decade ago, McCrea said, this would have been difficult to imagine.

Today's concussion research is almost elemental: the foundation upon which future scientific breakthroughs will be based. Collins and his group in Pittsburgh have identified six different clinical profiles for concussion, and they often overlap: vestibular, ocular-motor, cognitive, post-traumatic migraines, cervical, and anxiety/mood issues. The science of concussion has recognized that these brain injuries home in on the specific vulnerabilities of a particular brain. "Concussion fights dirty," Collins said. "It decompensates certain systems of the brain. Patients with a history of carsickness are more likely to have vestibular issues following a concussion. Patients with a history of migraine are more likely to have migraine. People with a history of lazy eye are more likely to have ocular dysfunction. Patients with anxiety are more likely to be anxious, and patients with learning disabilities are more likely to have cognitive issues following a concussion. The point is, we're starting to find that it may not be how hard you get hit in the head but what you bring to the table when you get hit in the head."

Meanwhile, treatment is becoming streamlined. An NCAA study from two decades ago showed that for 42 percent of concussed players, there was no symptom-free waiting period to return to play. Half of those players returned to play a day or two *before* concussion symptoms abated. That's the worst possible thing to do after a concussion. But a joint study between the NCAA and the Department of Defense, conducted between 2014 and 2017, showed that 99 percent of concussed patients had a symptom-free waiting period before returning to play of more than one day, and 40 percent had a symptom-free waiting period of more than seven days. That means concussed players are being withheld for longer than their period of cerebral vulnerability.

As researchers and scientists tackle what may be an existential question for football—How can brain trauma be mitigated in contact sports?—so too does the business world. Riddell's newest technology involves a Carbon 3-D helmet, with the interior fitted to each specific head size and shape and then printed from a 3-D printer. Five years from now, Riddell hopes to be offering off-the-rack helmets tuned specifically to each player. The NCAA's headache task force has focused on assertive and quick treatment from the moment after a concussion to avoid long-term problems. And the most recent research says that the proper treatment after a concussion is not to simply rest—not to cocoon people in dark rooms and limit physical activity. More effective is targeted physical activity like walking, jogging, or light lifting that doesn't put the brain at risk.

This is an important scientific conversation. But perhaps even more important is the cultural conversation around concussion. After all, this is a sport in which an NFL player named Russell Allen, in a 2013 game with the Jacksonville Jaguars, took a big hit to the head and suffered a stroke on the field. Even more concerning was that Allen refused to come out of that game; he didn't want to lose his starting job. (He eventually did lose his job, when the Jaguars released him four months later.) This play-through-it mentality is simply part of the fiber of this ruthless sport. As Sills stood before the group of neuroscientists and athletic trainers, he essentially admitted as much. The data that the NFL compiled on head injuries compelled the competition committee to adopt a rule before the 2018 season that penalized any player for lowering his head to initiate a hit on an opponent with his helmet. No sooner did the preseason games begin in August 2018 than the cries came from fans and players alike about these restrictive new rules. "A lot of people described that as the end of football, said it would be unwatchable, said it would be the worst thing that ever happened," Sills said. Plenty more people said it would be the most significant and positive rule change the NFL ever made. The outcry quieted to an occasional murmur; players and fans adapted, as they always do.

As emotional as major rule changes can be—*They're sissifying football!*—they are essential to the sport's survival. For decades, the NFL's own entertainment arm, NFL Films, released wildly popular VHS tapes that glorified these types of hits. The films had names like *Big Blocks and King Size Hits*, *Bone Crunchers*, and *Thunder and Destruction*. Most of the plays in these videos would result in flags, perhaps in ejection, today. "No one watches those videos [of big helmet-to-helmet hits] today and says, 'Wow, that's a great hit,'" Sills said.

Those "king size" hits, however, may not even be the central issue facing football. Big helmet-to-helmet hits can be legislated out of the game, or at least minimized, as the NFL has attempted to do in recent years. But what about repetitive subconcussive impacts that football players in certain positions, specifically on the offensive line and defensive line, experience on every single play? These head impacts are smaller, but they build up over time. The truth is, scientists don't have a great understanding of risk factors for how CTE develops. The majority of CTE cases have extensive exposure to both repetitive subconcussive head impacts as well as multiple instances of concussion. The prevailing hypothesis now among scientists is that players who experience those repetitive subconcussive head impacts carry more risk for developing CTE and more severe CTE than those having a history of concussion. In other words, having thousands (or even tens of thousands) of smaller impacts to the brain during a career might be more dangerous than a few massive impacts to the brain. This is what becomes the biggest threat to the future of football. It may be difficult to take the big head impacts out of the game, but it can be done. It feels nearly impossible to take smaller head impacts out of the game. America is addicted to the National Football League. But would America's addiction be transferred to the National Flag Football League?

The frontier of concussion research may determine that future. And part of that future is currently being worked on in a drab concrete office building in an industrial park near Minneapolis. Prevent Biometrics, founded in 2015, believes that to solve the concussion problem, we must first accurately measure impacts to the head. The company invented a smart mouth guard that does just that. There have been attempts to make head-impact monitors as part of the helmet, or embedded in skull caps, or as sensors attached to the skin, or implanted on headbands. The problem was that in high-impact collisions, these monitors would move around and the accuracy wasn't good.

Since upper teeth are rigidly connected to the human skull, any skull impact can be extrapolated accurately by measuring force felt in the teeth. The Prevent Biometrics mouth guards are equipped with a flexible circuit board embedded with a battery, a microprocessor, Bluetooth capabilities, and LED lights (which illuminate when a worrisome head impact is detected). This mouth guard doesn't measure or diagnose concussions. It measures head impacts. The sensors measure how much the teeth moved, then they triangulate that data to show how much the center of gravity in the head moved. Through an app, a coach or trainer has the ability to monitor head impacts in real time. Players who've experienced too many head impacts or a particularly hard hit can be red-flagged quickly. A head impact lasts .02 seconds, or twenty milliseconds. That's a tenth of a blink of an eye: Far too quick to diagnose from observation only. The mouth guard serves like a blood pressure monitor for head impacts.

Just as important as flagging vulnerable brains on the field will be the reams of accurate head-impact data that can be combined with clinical results and sent to researchers. One of the most stunning parts of the infancy of concussion research is that experts have little idea exactly how many sport-related concussions occur in the United States annually. Estimates range from 300,000 to 3.8 million. Put another way: We don't know within an order of magnitude how big a problem concussion really is.

Unfortunately, all this—the hundreds of millions of dollars for concussion research, the massive media and political attention, the cutting-edge biomedical technologies—doesn't mean paradigm-shifting results are coming anytime soon. As exciting as it can be when you hear people like Allen Sills talk about improvements over the past several years, that excitement gets quickly tempered when scientists talk about how long it will be until this research can actually make a major difference. "It wouldn't shock me," Adam Bartsch, the chief science officer at Prevent Biometrics, said, in a statement echoed by every serious scientist I've spoken with, "if we're at the start of a thirty-year learning curve."

Zac Easter's journal, July 12, 2015

Therapy is going all right, cognitively I'm still slow and physically my dizziness doesn't seem much better . . . My emotions still just seem fucked up. I've been stressed w/ all this stuff and I don't really feel like doing much. Been sitting around the house a lot and its hard for me to want to go out and do much. Its just easier for me when I avoid everyone. I wish there was a magic pill for me. I do just get sick of living this life and I try to stay motivated but its all self motivation from brain tremors. Everything I'm motivated to do has still yet to be accomplished. I wish I could put a finger on what is wrong with me. Its either from the concussions or Im just bat shit crazy. Im tired of feeling emotionless or too many emotions. Im trying to find a new hobby but nothing really quite makes me want to do it. Tomorrow I meet w/ Spooner about everything to me, there's just NO way those concussions didn't change me. I think I might just donate my brain and let them figure it out. I talked with my boss today and he understands why I cant work. IDK I might have to go on medical disability for right now. Every day has been a struggle for years. Hopefully this will stop. I want to be like everyone else.

THE NEXT DAY was the last time Zac met with Spooner. After that, he just quit. Gave up. Lost hope. Spooner never heard from him again, and he didn't hear anything about what happened to Zac until five months later, when he got a call from another doctor who'd been working with Zac. It was a call that stopped Spooner right in his tracks, that hit him in the gut harder than any hit he'd experienced on the football field. "You don't like to fail as a doctor," Spooner would later say. "It pissed me off—*God, what did I miss?*"

Despite everything, though, Spooner would still love football. During his sports medicine fellowship at Camp Pendleton, he'd be on the sidelines at Chargers games, learning as much as he could. Junior Seau had retired a couple of years before, but he was still the most revered Charger of all time, and the stands were filled with fans wearing Chargers jerseys emblazoned with Seau's number, 55. Spooner also worked as a sideline doctor on Friday nights at Oceanside High School, the same high school Seau had attended, just a few miles southwest of Camp Pendleton's main gate. It was on May 2, 2012, less than a year after Spooner completed the navy fellowship, when he heard the news that shocked the football world: Seau had shot himself in the chest at his beachfront home in Oceanside. Almost a year later, Seau's family released the findings from the National Institute of Neurological Disorders and Stroke, to whom they had donated his brain. Seau's brain had tested positive for CTE.

A few years later, after Spooner's tour in Afghanistan, after he joined a medical practice in a Des Moines suburb, his nine-year-old son announced to his parents that he wanted to play football. Spooner knew about the scientific studies that indicated playing tackle football before age twelve can be tied to an increased risk of brain problems later in life. And he'd read about former NFL players who recently joined up with the Boston-based Concussion Legacy Foundation for a new parent education initiative, Flag Football Under 14, that dissuades parents from allowing their kids to play tackle football before age fourteen.

Spooner and his wife tried to talk their son out of football—*Why not soccer? Soccer would be safer!* But it was not as easy a parental diktat as you would think. All their son's friends were playing football. Spooner wanted his son to have the same social experience that he'd had in his own childhood. He didn't want to protect his son so much that all he did was stay in the house and play video games. So in third grade, his son played in a flag football league that had the boys wear soft-shell helmets, a slightly more aggressive version of flag football that focused heavily on fundamentals. In fourth grade, his son was supposed to play flag football in full pads—one season to get used to the equipment—then by fifth grade, he would move on to padded, tackle football.

The potential consequences of football wore on Spooner. Plus his son was small compared with other football players. For a year, he kept hammering home to his son the risks of football, but he wanted his son to make the decision on his own. Finally, the boy decided to play soccer instead. Spooner knows soccer is a sport with substantial concussion risk, with headers and plenty of incidental contact. But U.S. Soccer banned headers in youth soccer in 2016, and Spooner took solace in the fact that soccer concussions tend to be freak injuries, as opposed to in football, with concussions and subconcussive hits seeming to be a natural part of the game.

Still, his son could have decided on football, and Spooner would have lived with that.

"We should have a healthy fear of concussions and treat them appropriately," Spooner said. "But I'd hate to have them feared so much that we start keeping kids from being physically active and from enjoying things like sports."

"Here's the thing," Spooner continued. "I don't want to put my kid in a bubble. I want him to experience what it's like to be on a team. That's a powerful experience, whether it's a football team or a military squad or whatever team you're on. He knows there's a chance he could get hurt. Parents and coaches know there's a chance [kids] could get hurt. No guarantees. I know it can happen with anything, but something about the football stigma even has me spooked. If he got a concussion [in football] and it's a bad one, I may regret it. But if everyone is educated on the risks, and there are significant benefits, and if the vast majority of people who go through it have vast benefits, I'm just going to let it go. See how it goes. It can happen in soccer. It can happen on your bike. It can happen any other place. Sometimes you gotta trust fate, I guess."

Spooner has another son, a tough kid a few years younger than his firstborn. Spooner knows the family is going to have this same discussion and this same concern. The doctor isn't sure which way the choice will go.

EIGHT

The Reckoning

Zac Easter's journal, June 30, 2015

The past week I've been stressed out from not getting enough sleep and the Wellbutrin makes me feel weird. I took it for a while and stopped once I noticed it was giving me insomnia and actually making me depressed. I'm still going to speech therapy and PT. Dr. Spooner is also sending me to a mental health psych because I might be a little mentally ill. Personally I wouldn't be surprised. I've been to the Dr. so many damn times over my life and they always say my head is fine. So maybe I'm missing a screw lol. IDK I'm open to going down that path and figure it out. I just know I can't sustain the life I'm living so I'm willing to see anyone at this point. I'm tired of having to eat healthy, work out several times a day, or use drugs/alcohol to feel normal around people. If only people could see the world through my eyes and see the mental battle I fight every day. Only God knows whats it like because he has been the only one to guide me through the light of darkness and into the brightness of the future. I had quite a few thoughts of suicide over the past week, but I told that Zac to go fuck himself. I'm not giving up and I know God is still on my side watching my back from letting my mind slip into temptation. Either way this weekend should be fun. Fourth of July is usually a nice [break] from reality for me.

THE SUMMER OF 2015 was filled with stops and starts for Zac. There were moments of hope when he felt on top of the world, when he felt one of these doctors would finally lead him to that magic pill. He recorded his emotions and his coping strategies, and when he was feeling at his highest, he'd scribble down aspirational lists of his life goals. To his family, he'd often pretend that every-thing was normal, doing things like going to a gun show with his dad and his younger brother, Levi, and showing up for family meals. But there were also deepening moments of despair; at one point, he sat down at his computer and started typing out a suicide note. One night, he even resolved to kill himself. "Thank god I was to drunk one night and passed out while doing it," he wrote. At the gun show, he attempted to tell his dad and younger brother what was going on inside his brain. "It was awkward when I tried telling them a little about whats wrong w/ my head. I ended up dropping it."

After his twenty-fourth birthday in June, when he revealed the depth of his brain issues to his parents, his mother did everything she could to save him. She insisted on going to some of his therapist appointments. When she was there with him, Zac would get angry and embarrassed. He hated talking in front of his mom about his emotions and drug abuse and how much he had struggled just to get through school. When the therapist asked about things like abusing Adderall to get over his social anxiety, Zac's face got flushed. His heart raced. The doctor noted Zac's anxiety at his questions, and he backed off.

Every time he left these appointments, Zac felt lost and confused. One time, he walked into the parking lot and for several minutes couldn't find his car. "I drove home in one of those trances I get in and damn near almost hit a car and took a bunch of wrong turns," Zac wrote in his journal. "Shits starting to get fucked up for me. IDK . . . I'm going nuts lol."

Zac was sleepless and on edge; too much Adderall will do that. Again and again, he pledged to quit, but he kept coming back to it. When some buddies invited him to Lake of the Ozarks in Missouri for a weekend of partying, he declined: "I just feel super avoidant and I don't feel like being around anyone." Instead of hanging out with friends, he'd stay in his room and masturbate for hours; hypersexual behavior can be a complication associated with head injuries. While his friends were at the lake, Zac finally relented with a girl who'd been bugging him to hang out. (Ali and Zac had been in this hybrid intense-but-casual semi-relationship for months, but they weren't official—so why not?) The girl came over to his place, and they had sex all night. "It was nice to just fuck for like 5 hrs and not think about my brain," Zac wrote. "Overall the sex was great and was a nice release from the normal jerking off every night . . . Fuck it. Pussy was nice."

The next day, Zac went to his parents' house for dinner. He was exhausted—he had been up with the girl until 5:00 a.m. and awoken at 8:00 a.m.—so he popped a few Adderall. As soon as he walked into his parents' house, his mood shifted to anger. One reason was that his brother Levi was having friends over, and Zac didn't want to be around them. More urgently, though, his medical records had been mailed to his parents' house, and they had looked through them. "I kinda tried to be ok about it but inside I wanted to freak out and I felt like its not their problem its mine," Zac wrote. "I know they just want to help. I honestly feel like its not their business to know about all my problems. I still feel insecure about letting them know." He told his mom that he didn't want her to attend his doctor appointments anymore, and that he had signed a document saying health-care information couldn't be released to anyone but him. She thought Zac was hiding something. "I kind of snapped a little and told her its just whats best for me." He hated that his problems were putting more stress on the family. So he made up an excuse to leave and drive back to Des Moines.

Back home, he couldn't sleep, so he jacked off until 6:00 a.m. He woke up a few hours later to go to lunch with his grandparents. He was late. His eyes were bloodshot. Zac barely spoke during the meal. It was awkward: "I felt anxiety and depressed the whole time," he later wrote.

As Zac walked out to his car, his younger brother, Levi, followed him. He asked if Zac was OK. He asked if he was still taking his antidepressants. "If you need to talk," Levi told him, "just call me."

"I told him Im ok and it's just I haven't slept much lately," Zac wrote in his journal. "Really I want to tell someone that I'm a wreck inside."

Zac drove home and popped some more Adderall. He stayed up all night researching concussions on his computer.

"I need to keep control of what I still can in my life," Zac wrote. "I also hate how I feel like I might snap any moment on someone . . . I'm willing to do whatever it takes to get help. I just hope I'm not fully loosing my mind."

    * * *

Zac Easter's journal, August 5, 2015

Oops sorry its been awhile since my last entry. Everything has been going about the same though. Still faced with daily depression and anxiety about stupid shit. Right now grandpa is in the hospital and he almost wasn't able to pull through. Jake bought a puppy husky and that has been helping me with the stress. I still haven't been working or looking for work.

I got put on Zoloft and my new psychiatrist seems to know his meds. I'm still fighting the side effects. Sleep has been dismal and I've still been going to speech therapy and PT. It sounds like they really aren't on my side anymore and they want me to be focusing on my mood disorder. I can't really blame them. I have been fucked up with depression the past few weeks. I've been going out more but using more drugs. Smoked pot a few times, rolled on Molly and now I got some coke. All that plus Adderall fuck it! It's the only way I feel normal. I'm going to try getting a PT job untill the Zoloft kicks in. IDK what to do about a career right now. I'm just sick of living life how I'm living it so I'm trying to get right. I wouldn't mind traveling. My confidence is a little low now that I know I'm not that smart. Oh well hopefully I can get some sleeping pills to help me sleep and I think that'll help with the depression. My impulse control has been a little better but I still cant get myself to want to be around ppl. Sometimes I just feel like snapping."

IT WAS THE end of summer, and time was running short with Ali. She'd always been a go-getter, and she was moving to Cleveland to attend law school at Case Western Reserve. Why did things shift between Zac and Ali? Maybe it was that Zac's brain and mood issues were worsening. Maybe it was because Ali was the only person Zac felt that he could be his authentic, vulnerable, damaged self with. Or maybe it was that this on-again, off-again romance now had a very serious deadline, with Ali moving almost seven hundred miles away for a life that would be consumed with studies and tests and internships for the next three years. Whatever the reason, that summer—as Zac was grappling with his ongoing problems with his brain and mental health—something was changing about their relationship. Ali has always had a bit of a savior complex, forever motivated by the urge to help others; so perhaps it was fate that during Zac's rapid descent, their relationship went from on-again, off-again to fully on.

Zac was struggling. His impulse control was shot. He couldn't stop binge eating unless he popped an Adderall or two; the fitness freak had turned into a junk-food obsessive. His parents checked his bank account and were shocked at how much he was spending, including dozens of debit card transactions a day at convenience stores. "I used to be a tight ass and all about money, but now I just find myself spending all my money and money that I don't even have," Zac wrote. Over the span of three months, he burned through about $10,000 and had nothing to show for it. He couldn't sleep. He was frequently dizzy. A guy who just a couple of years before was the fitness star of his military unit now stopped, out of breath and dizzy, only a couple of minutes into a jog. "I don't know if I have that brain decise that people talk about," Zac wrote, "or if I really am crazy."

One night, Zac overheard one of his roommates say he was a weirdo. Zac was crushed. By this point, with his bank account dwindling, he couldn't afford rent for much longer, so he figured he'd end up moving back to his parents' house. He'd gotten a doc-tor's note for a medical discharge from the military. "Good thing! I hate the fucking Army," wrote Zac, tossing away those dreams of becoming an Army Ranger. Instead of chasing the army badass dream he'd always wanted, his goals were more modest. He was interviewing for jobs as a restaurant host at several Des Moines res-taurants: a chic Italian place called Centro, an elegant, James Beard Award–nominated establishment called Bistro Montage, a rowdy New Orleans–inspired roadhouse called Buzzard Billy's. None of the jobs came through. In his journal, he scribbled down other ideas for work: staining decks, or landscaping, or maybe a newspaper delivery route. In the meantime, he could prepare for the GMAT and start the process of getting into graduate school. Maybe he could even follow Ali and go to business school at Case Western Reserve University's Weatherhead School of Management. "Its all part of the success story," Zac wrote next to this modest to-do list in his journal. With Ali, he gave himself permission to dream.

Nothing seemed to be going right. Except, that is, things with Ali. Previously, their relationship had been a casual thing, which meant they'd be together when Ali was home but go their own ways when she was at school. They hadn't wanted to be in a long-distance relationship when Ali was an undergrad in Kentucky and Zac was in Iowa. And they didn't want the small-town rumor mill to chatter about them. So they talked and they texted, but they never discussed who either of them was dating, and they never turned their relationship into anything official—never called each other boyfriend or girlfriend, never checked the "in a relationship" box on Facebook, never overtly held hands when they were out with a group of high school friends. But when winter or summer vacations came, they'd fall back into their routine like nothing had changed: to the bar with friends, then disappearing together for a "rum and Coke." The time when they were apart had an unexpected effect: It made them best friends, not just lovers. "We're both good at compartmentalizing," Ali said. "But in the back of my head, I always knew who I'd be with." Zac's mother approved; she knew there was something between these two, and she started to think of Ali as the daughter she never had. Ali's parents and friends approved, too. She had always dated "douchebags," as Zac called them, but here was Zac, this good, fun-loving country boy who was loyal to those he loved and curious about the world.

That summer, as they got closer, they went to Lake Ahquabi and lay in the grass. They half joked about who would be in their wedding party, and what their children would be like. When Zac spoke about going to business school, Ali encouraged him; both had big goals, and they believed they'd achieve them together. They shared a playlist on Spotify with songs they loved. One was "My Escape" by the Canadian band Ravenscode, with haunting lyrics about not letting a loved one "slip away," and needing someone "till the very end."

There were just five days before Ali was to leave for law school. Later, she would refer to this time as "the perfect week." On Monday, she and Zac met at Gray's Lake. They sat at a picnic table and gazed at Des Moines's skyline. They went to the movie theater to see *Trainwreck*, the Amy Schumer comedy. They laughed and giggled the whole time. At one point, Zac reached over and grabbed Ali's hand. This was a big deal: an expression of love, in public, while sober. They got some drinks at a bar near the mall, then they went back to Zac's place.

On Tuesday, they went for another walk around Gray's Lake. Neither of them wanted to hang out with anyone else; they didn't want to have to pretend anymore. They went to a place called Zombie Burger + Drink Lab, a zombie-themed burger joint. They ordered two Undead Elvis burgers: a hamburger patty topped with peanut butter, fried bananas, bacon, American cheese, mayonnaise, and a soft egg. They walked around Des Moines's East Village in the shadow of the state capitol building, then they dropped by a martini lounge. They were the only two at the bar. They talked about life for two hours—about religion, about law school, about Zac's struggling brain, about politics. Ali had interned for Democratic US Senator Tom Harkin, and she tried to guide Zac toward the left side of the political spectrum. And they talked about football. He'd spent a lot of that summer reflecting about the sport, and the many things it had brought to his life. The good things, like the camaraderie of the team, the connection with his father and brothers, the excitement of playing in a game, the thrill of rooting for his favorite NFL team. And the bad things, like however the game had contributed to this crazy thing that was going on in his brain. Ali was the only one he spoke with about this. He never brought up his ambivalence about football to his family. "Zac would always tell me he got a lot out of football," Ali said. "He also felt like it was expected for him to play. He didn't want to take himself out of games. At times, he really did still love the game. At times, he hated it. He'd say to me, 'I don't even know why I played football that long, but I couldn't have quit.'"

Whenever he confided thoughts like this to her, he always made an addendum: "Don't tell my family." So many of his familial ties revolved around football. He didn't want his parents and brothers and others to know his struggles with his brain betraying him, and how he suspected football as a cause, perhaps the main cause. Part of it, Ali suspected, was a sense of shame—that Zac felt his issues were evidence that he hadn't lived up to the ideal definition of what it meant to be a man. The test of manhood that he always thought football represented had come to represent his own failure. Now, he couldn't even hold down a job.

The next day, Ali finished up at her summer job at the Express clothing store at the mall, and a group of girls from work took her out for a goodbye dinner. Zac joined them. Hanging with people he didn't know, feeling socially awkward, Zac slammed several drinks in succession, becoming really, really drunk in a flash. Ali got pissed. She texted him: "I hate you, but I love you." They hopped around to a few bars. Ali made sure Zac got home safely that night; once he got home, she cared for him as he threw up from all the alcohol.

"I've been in love with you for five years," Zac told her, drunk. "I don't get why you can't see this."

"Zac," Ali soothed him, "why don't we have this conversation when we're sober?" She didn't want them to have a big, emotional conversation only to have him forget it the next day.

When Zac woke up the next morning, he had a massive head-ache and few memories of the night before. "What did I do?" Zac asked Ali. They went to get their cars. But both had been parked illegally, and their cars had been towed. They laughed at their bad luck. Before Ali left to go to the Iowa State Fair with her parents, she met Zac's gaze and said: "We should talk later." That night, on Thursday, August 13, 2015, they met at Gray's Lake. It had been a steamy Iowa summer day, but by the time they were dodging cyclists and joggers as they walked around the lake, the temperature had, mercifully, dipped below eighty degrees. For an hour, they circled the lake and dodged the elephant in the room. Then, Ali told Zac what he'd said the night before: that he'd been in love with her for five years. "Yes," he said. "It's all true."

Finally, it was out there. And it was out there while they were sober. They went back to Zac's place and talked over their options. One, they could date each other exclusively despite Ali leaving for law school in two days. Two, they could stop seeing each other entirely. Three, they could keep up with this in-between crap.

Zac thought it over for the night.

The next morning, a day before Ali left, he turned to her in bed: "OK," he said, "let's do it." They spent the entire day together. They watched one of their favorite television shows, *Shameless*, a dark TV comedy about a dysfunctional family in Chicago, and *House of Lies*, another TV comedy about a group of cutthroat management consultants. It was August 14. They made their relationship public—told friends, told family, announced it on Facebook.

The next day, August 15, Ali left Indianola and drove to Cleveland to begin law school.

"And right after I left," she said, "it started to go downhill."

Zac Easter's journal, September 5, 2015

Just got back from spending some more time with Ali [in Cleveland]. IDK if I've told you but me and Ali are dating now. We've been super tight for years and now we're already saying we love each other. IDK how I feel about yet. She still seems emotionally unavailable and its killing my own emotions. I just don't think shes very aware of what she does. She wont tell me how she feels and I know she feels just as vulnerable as me. IDK Im falling for her hard and I really just don't want to get myself hurt. IDK if I can be with though when I'm this insecure. She has helped me get myself more motivated, plus Im just out of money and I need to start working again. I got enough for one more months rent but after that Im screwed. I havent told Ali that the real reason I cant come up is because Im broke. I still feel like shes more distant than ever . . . I think Im just going to stop chasing her and slowly start to break myself off from this attachment. I just cant do it right now.

Other than that, my depression seems to be getting worse. Ive been taking Zoloft and Adderall now for a month and a half and I don't really feel better, if anything I feel worse. I keep having crazy mood swings and Im just not sure where my emotions are and Im so sick of it. I need more therapy and I want to get help. I also need to go talk with my parents.

I'm scared if I can't get help or feel better I may want to just end it all. As in suicide. Im just so tired of feeling so shitty and anxious. I had a job interview, two of them and its hard for me to not have panic attacks. It seems like I still cant get over my anxiety. IDK lifes just a bitch. Im try to forget about that fact that Im mentally ill and that I might have a traumatic brain disorder. I plan on going home tonight so hopefully I'll be able to talk to my rents a little more. I might even move home next month if I cant get some income coming in. I honestly just want to move and be with Ali, but I don't think that will happen when I need to start separating myself as it is. I feel like my drinking problem is starting to come back so Im going to try and not drink this weekend. And also try to not spend money. I just got my Adderall script and started snorting it right away! Im going to try and leave it home when I go home so I don't use it all. Physically my heart rate is still always nuts whether I'm Adderall or not. I'm trying to work out but its just getting harder each day. So yeah I guess that's an update for now.

ONE SEPTEMBER NIGHT in Indianola, Zac forced himself to go to a party at a high school friend's house in honor of another friend who had just graduated from the United States Military Academy at West Point and was working toward becoming an Army Ranger. It had been a couple of months since Zac had seen Nick Haworth, his close friend since childhood and a former high-school football teammate. Haworth congratulated Zac—he'd seen his name in the newspaper recently for making honor roll at Grand View University during his final semester. "It seemed like he got his shit together," Haworth said. There was a video from that night of Zac in a beer-chugging contest with friends. He seemed joyful, his old happy self.

The three young men—Zac, Haworth, and Lance Parker, the friend who was back from West Point—took their beers and headed to the back deck for some catch-up time between good buddies. They sat on a table while Haworth lit a cigarette. Zac wasn't too talkative. Then, after a while, he started speaking up.

"I'm kind of going through some shit," Zac said. "I've been out of work."

He hadn't worked in two months, he told his friends. His headaches were constant. He had just moved back in with his parents. He could no longer afford rent. As he sipped from his beer at the party, he told his friends that he hadn't mentioned these struggles before because he didn't want to burden other people with his problems.

"I think I have this thing called chronic traumatic encephalopathy," Zac told them. Haworth had no idea what he was talking about. Zac detailed the turn his life had taken: depression, head-aches, mood swings. At first, doctors had told him about postcon-cussion syndrome. Then, they mentioned this much scarier disease. Zac told them that this was the disease that Chris Benoit, the leg-endary Canadian professional wrestler, had contracted after a con-cussion-filled wrestling career. Benoit had murdered his wife and seven-year-old son at their home in 2007 before hanging himself. Posthumous tests showed that his brain was so severely damaged that it looked like the brain of an eighty-something-year-old suf-fering from Alzheimer's disease.

Zac's two friends were speechless. The next day, they met up again to talk about Zac. "Man," one friend said to the other, "it sounds like his brain is turning to fucking mush."

THAT WHOLE FALL, everything seemed dark to Zac. The weather was gloomy, cloudy, rainy. It felt like the whole world had turned black. His mood matched the skies. Before he moved back in with his parents, he'd lock himself in his room and drink, sometimes appearing in the living room for ten minutes wearing sweatpants and an expressionless look before disappearing back into his room. His roommates were concerned. Things only got worse. His family knew about Zac's struggles now, but to his parents and brothers it appeared he was getting better. In September, to celebrate Zac's older brother's birthday, they all went to Bensink Farms Hunting Preserve in the nearby town of Pleasantville. Zac seemed like his old self. He posted a photo to Snapchat that day with the caption: Time to shoot some shit.

Pheasant season was to begin on Halloween, Zac's father's birthday. The Easter men planned to go hunting on their grandpa's farm. The night before, Zac's dad gave him simple instructions:

"You bring your boots. I'll bring your gun." It was chilly and rainy on Halloween morning when Zac pulled up in Big Red to the family farm. He was wearing shorts and tennis shoes. "I thought, *What in the fuck, you dumbass?*" Myles Easter Sr. recalled later.

"It's fricking freezing out," Myles Sr. told his middle son. "You're gonna get sick."

Zac opened a rear door of his Mazda and started looking around the back seat.

"What are you looking for, your boots?" Myles Sr. asked him.

"No, you got my boots, Dad," Zac replied. "I'm looking for my gun."

Myles Easter shook his head. He had told Zac this the night before—*You bring your boots. I'll bring your gun.*—and Zac had gotten it mixed up. That wasn't like Zac. Myles Sr. had been skeptical the past several months when Zac told the family about his problems with his memory and his brain, and the concussions from football that might have been the cause. The explanation felt like an excuse to Myles Sr. He figured Zac was a twenty-four-year-old kid struggling to adjust to adulthood. This brain thing? It was just an excuse for him becoming a bit of a fuckup, like plenty of twenty-something young men do as they are trying to find their way in life. But on this day, Daddy Myles started to see a different and scarier version of his middle son.

They walked in the open field. Zac's tennis shoes got soaked and covered in mud. He didn't seem to mind. Myles Easter noticed a hollow look in his son's eyes: distant, empty, a pair of dark holes in a disconnected countenance that didn't resemble his Zac. The Easter men found a raccoon hiding in a hole near a fence. One of the dogs was trying to get it. Zac walked up and shot the raccoon. He displayed no emotion. To Myles Sr., this expressionless young man didn't seem one bit like his middle son. It awakened the father to a realization.

"When we were walking in the field," Myles Sr. said, "I thought, *Maybe there's more to this.*"

IT WAS A chilly day in November 2015. Friday the 13th, of all days. Cloudy, of course. Ali had been gone for nearly three months. Early that morning, Zac texted her while she slept: "I'm sorry you fell in love with a guy with a ducked up brain." At some point after sending that text to Ali, Zac started drinking from a bottle of Jack Daniel's in his childhood bedroom. His mother had found empty bottles of liquor whenever she came in to clean his room: "Zac, did you drink all this?" she'd asked. So he'd started to hide the bottles from her.

Now, Big Red was swerving around the wide suburban boulevards of West Des Moines late that morning, with Zac at the wheel. He was shit-faced. He knew Ali was in class. Shortly before 10:00 a.m., he texted her while driving: "Can you call me when you get out of class? I'm in hot water right now and idk what to do."

A couple of nights before, on Wednesday, Zac and Ali had gotten into a fight. Zac had said some mean things; she told him she needed a couple of days of not talking to him. It wasn't breaking up, not exactly, but for both of them, it kind of felt like it. For four hours that night, they didn't text each other. Then, a text from Zac popped up on Ali's phone: "Is it just me or does this seem kind of dumb? Lol" Then, another text from Zac, apologizing again: "Look you probably still hate me and I don't blame you. One bit. I won't lie to you and I'm not bs'ing you and just trying to get your attention. I'm not sure I'm doing well physically because weird things are happening my body." He texted her again: "Sounds crazy I know, but if there's one person I want to make things right with its you. I'm sorry for everything. There's no simple way of saying it and it doesn't even sound sincere like this. But some day I hope you find it in your heart to forgive."

Ali wrote a terse response: "Whats wrong" Followed by: "And I don't hate you. I hope your body is feeling better."

Zac didn't reply until the next morning, on Thursday: "Sorry I passed out last night, it was weird my heart was like off beat and my head was like having a seizure. Idk. It was fucked up and I couldn't move. It sounds a little dramatic now, but I felt I was dying or something haha that's why I texted you . . . Sorry though!!"

Another text from Zac: "Could you talk to me tonight? I don't want to guilt trip you and stuff. But your the only one who knows me and I really need someone to talk to."

ALI: Yeah we can talk later tonight. What time were you thinking?

ZAC: Idc I'm free all day/night.

ZAC, TWO HOURS LATER: Well shit, I forgot I had to do a family thing tonight until later. Don't worry about it. (Ali was still mad at him from their fight. But she knew he needed her. They worked out a time to talk.)

ZAC: Well I guess do you even want to talk? Lol idk I don't want to make you upset or mess with your feelings.

ALI: "You wont be—I won't let you lol I told you I'd be therr for you so just choose a time dudeeeeeeeee

He chose 10:00 p.m. Then, he texted her again: "Yeah but you don't have to worry about [it.]"

ALI: Zac stop. I told you we could talk.

ZAC: Well you make me feel like it's a hassle or that it's a burden lol

ALI: What have I said that makes you feel like that

ZAC: You haven't said it, but your texts and the way they are presented to me just kind of make me feel that way.

Ali was frustrated. Her boyfriend's mood was all over the place. She tried not to let her frustration show: "If it was a hassle I wouldn't have said yes so don't worry about that."

It was a little after 10:00 p.m. Zac didn't pick up when she called. She texted him again: "Hellllllooo Zachary? Lol just call me when you want to talk."

He didn't pick up. He didn't pick up all night. Ali was worried, but his mood had been like a Ping-Pong ball for months. She assumed he'd passed out.

The next morning, on Friday, November 13, a text from Zac popped up on Ali's phone at 5:40 a.m.: "Sorry about last night."

Ali: "What happened to ya?"

No response. Ali didn't know it, but around that time is when Zac started drinking. He was hearing voices inside his head.

Ali texted him again at 9:32 a.m. "Look I meant it when I said I wanted a few days to myself to clear my head but I also meant it when I said I'd always be there for you, even during that time. If you need to talk then we will talk you just gotta let me know when. I'm done with class at noon, so if you still need me we can talk then or later on—up to you."

Ali didn't know it at the time, but Zac was driving drunk around West Des Moines.

"Yes I still need to talk," Zac texted. "Can you call me when you get out of class? I'm in hot water right now and idk what to do"

As soon as she got out of class and saw Zac's text, Ali called him. He was slurring his words, crying, talking about having lost all hope, apologizing for being a fuckup. Ali was scared, but she talked him down, like she always did. She convinced him to stop at a gas station to get him off the road. He hung up on her. He got a Gatorade.

"Do not leave," Ali texted him at 11:27 a.m.

She coaxed him into a nearby Jimmy John's to sober up.

She texted him again: "I'm not trying to be mean or make you feel like shit but I'm worried about you and have already lost my best friend to drunk driving. I'm not gonna be ok if I lose you too so just think of that."

They talked. She soothed him. She could hear his voice calm down. She texted him: "Idk if I did, but I hope I helped." He texted her back. She could feel the guilt and the shame through his words: "You did well babe. I'm sorry"

Back at home, in his bedroom, next to the Muhammad Ali poster that read: Impossible Is Nothing, his laptop was open to a thirty-nine-page Microsoft Word document titled "Concussions: My Silent Struggle." He'd created the document five months earlier. "My last wishes," it began. The final revision was made that day, November 13, 2015.

Then came a strange request from Zac. He asked what Ali's email address was. He already knew her email address—they'd emailed each other how many times over the years?—but she texted it to him anyway.

ZAC: You found another guy yet?
ALI: Of course not Zac
ZAC: K
ALI: I'm serious. Have you found another girl?
ZAC: No

ALI: Why are you mad
ZAC: I'm not. Your single do as you please
ALI: Zac I'm well aware. But I have no desire to be with anyone.
ZAC: Ok

Zac promised he wouldn't drive. Ali went into a meeting about a law class. At some point later in the afternoon, Zac texted her: "I'm home now. Don't worry about it lol thanks for the help though!"

ALI: Zac. You promised you weren't gonna drive.
ZAC: Ok sorry Alison. For everything. Idk what's happening to me, but I'm sorry I brought you into it.
ALI: Don't be sorry you brought me into it. I told you I'd always be there for you. I just want you to get better.
ZAC: Idk if there is better for ppl like me.
ALI: There is. You just need a little extra reminding
ZAC: I love you so much it's stupid. I'm sorry you fell in love with a guy with a ducked up brain.
ALI: You can't choose who you fall in love with. You just fall in love.
ZAC: Like I said before. If anything happens to be just by a chance of luck. Tell my family everything.

This sounded ominous. It was getting close to evening in Iowa. Zac grabbed the .40-caliber pistol he'd given his dad for Father's Day, got in Big Red, and pulled out of his parents' driveway. He drove up the hill and then down to the intersection, and he turned left onto the pavement. A couple of miles down the road, he took a right into Lake Ahquabi State Park. He'd had so many great memories at this lake. This would not be one of them.

Zac opened the Facebook app on his phone. He typed out a post: "Dear friends and family, If your reading this than God bless the times we've had together. Please forgive me. I'm taking the selfish road out. Only God understands what I've been through. No good times will be forgotten and I will always watch over you. Please if anything remember me by the person I am not by my actions. I will always watch over you! Please, please, don't take the easy way out like me. Fist pumps for Jesus and fist pumps for me. Party on wayne!!;)"

This wasn't just ominous; this was a very public suicide note. All around Indianola and Des Moines, friends and family saw Zac's post and panicked. *Where is Zac?* Zac's phone started buzzing, buzzing, buzzing. He didn't pick up. Ali called again and again. No reply. Nobody knew where he was. At 5:36 p.m., his first college roommate, Jake Powers, texted him: "Hey what're you up to bud?" No reply. The sun had dipped over the horizon on the other side of the Y-shaped lake. Leaves lay in heaps on the fringe of the woods. The gusty November winds died down as the sun sank, but there was still a chill in the air. Zac took out his phone and snapped a picture of the lake. He posted it to Snapchat, ignoring the frantic phone calls that were pouring into his phone. God bless America, he captioned the photo.

Ali called again.

Finally, Zac picked up. There was terror in his voice.

"I can't do this," he told her. "It's never going to get better."

A friend noticed the setting of Zac's Snapchat photo: Lake Ahquabi, just down the road from his family's house. Ali tried to soothe him: "Listen to the sound of my voice. Listen to the sound of my voice."

"I'm losing my mind," he cried into the phone. "This is it for me!" A police cruiser came speeding down the winding hill toward the lake, followed by another. "Ali, did you send these cops here?" Then, Zac's phone cut out.

Zac pointed the pistol at the darkened sky and fired a warning shot. Moments later, Myles Easter Sr. sped down the hill in his pickup. Men do not sit around and wait for life to happen to them; men get up and fix things. And Myles Easter knew he was needed to fix his son, right then. He jumped out of the truck and peered through the window of his son's car. He saw an empty six-pack of Coors Light, an empty bottle of Captain Morgan, and a pill bottle.

Floodlights illuminated Zac. He walked down the pier toward a wooden fishing hut out on the water. Zac's phone died. He didn't get the frantic and garbled text message Ali sent him at 6:12 p.m.: "Baby its my Winslow jist talk to me. I need to know you're okay.."

"Put your gun down!" the deputies shouted.

"Nope!" Zac yelled with an anguished laugh. "Not gonna do that!"

"Fuck it," Myles said to himself. "I can't let this happen. If he shoots me, he shoots me."

Zac's father sprinted past the sheriff's deputies and onto the pier.

"Dad, stop!"

"Zac, I'm coming," Myles said. "Put your gun down."

"Dad!" Zac shouted again. "Dad, stop!"

Zac disappeared into the fishing hut with his gun.

The door slammed shut behind him.

Seconds later his father reached the door. He opened it. He saw a sad, sick look on his son's face.

"Dad, I'm in trouble," Zac said quietly.

Myles Easter Sr. spoke gently. "I don't know what's going on, but we'll get this figured out. But we gotta get through this part right now. We're in deep shit. We can't make it any worse."

Zac handed over his gun. Slowly, his dad opened the door of the fishing hut. They walked up the pier to dry land, where deputies surrounded Zac and eased his wrists into handcuffs. An ambulance drove Zac to Des Moines, where he would be checked into Iowa Lutheran Hospital's psychiatric unit.

In Cleveland, Ali was still panicking. For sixty-two minutes, she had no idea if Zac was dead or alive. His final words to her before his phone died had sounded so flat, so final.

Finally, a text popped up on her phone. It was Zac's older brother: "They got him." Zac had been saved from himself.

NINE

The End

Email from Ali Epperson to Zac's older brother, Myles II, the day after his suicide attempt:

From: Alison Epperson <xxxx@gmail.com>
Date: Sat, Nov 14, 2015 at 1:20 PM
Subject: Zac history
To: Myles Easter <xxxx@gmail.com>

Hey—so I'm trying to remember and word all of it, but he's told me a lot so if I'm leaving anything out I'll try to pass it along as I remember (and I apologize for the random order of this e-mail. I'm just writing as it comes to me) . . .

Okay, so Zac first told me about all of the medical stuff this summer when I got home from school. He explained that all of it stemmed from all of the concussions he got in HS and that the consequences/symptoms were exacerbated because he never properly dealt with them and kept playing through them, etc. . . .

He also had these little brain spasms frequently. He described them as mini mini seizures. They'd last 1-5 seconds but would be a shooting intense pain in his head and he felt like he couldn't move during those seconds.

Like I said, he's talked to a bunch of doctors and therapists and he never felt like he was getting a real answer or any kind of consensus. Some of the possible things he was suffering from that he talked to doctors about was borderline bipolar disorder, borderline schizophrenia, and borderline personality disorder. (BPD was a big one for him that we talked about a lot) . . .

One thing that happened occasionally is he would get an overwhelmingly feeling of sadness or an off mood feeling that would come on suddenly and last a few hours without any explanation. One of the weekends he came to visit me, he came because he started having one of these episodes and wanted to get away from everyone at home. That's also the first weekend he skipped drill because the episode was that bad. He had another one on the drive here and then he had one while he was here . . .

It's true he had been drinking most nights. The past week and a half he'd been trying to push me away without saying that all of this was behind it until the past couple days when he all but admitted it. Wednesday night he texted me saying that he wasn't doing well and that his body felt physically off. He described it as his heart was off beat and he felt like he was having a mini seizure and couldn't move.

Yesterday he texted me during class and told me he really needed to talk and asked if I could call him after class. I got out of class an hour later and called him and he was drunk driving around WDM. I made him pull over and go get food at jimmy johns and wait there for awhile . . . I got him calmed down and we just talked about how he was gonna be able to beat all of this he just needed to stay committed to fighting it and getting help and needed to remember to call

me or his therapist or one of you all when he woke up in
the mood he did yesterday. He was still upset but a lot more
positive about it all.

Probably another 45 minutes went by and then he headed
home. I called him again after that and he said he was at
home and was feeling a little better and that he was just
gonna try to sleep for a couple hours.

Maybe two hours later I got a snap from him at lake
aquabi and then maybe an hour or hour and a half I saw the
status and called him.

When I called him he was bawling and just kept apologizing and saying he loved me but that he wasn't himself and
that he was going crazy, etc etc. He also mentioned hearing
voices again.

He hung up and then when I got him on the phone again
he was still crying. However, during this time he still knew
he was talking to me and was aware of what was going on.
He knew the cops were there, etc. I got him to calm down
very briefly and just listen to my voice but then he got flus-
tered again when he saw the cops get closer. Then he accused
me of helping the cops, but then he went back to apologizing
and said he already texted all of you and that he wanted his
brain donated to concussion research. He hung [up]. I got
him on the phone one last time for only about 30 seconds
and he was still really upset. After that he stopped answering
and then his phone just went straight to voicemail.

I know there's a lot more and I'm trying to remember and
piece it all together, but I'm emotionally exhausted after last
night so it's hard to remember. I'll keep sending you things
as I remember.

ON THE MORNING of Monday, November 16, 2015, less than seventy-two hours after he had pointed his .40-caliber pistol at the evening sky at Lake Ahquabi State Park and fired, Zac was sitting across the table from his mother at the IHOP next to a Walmart Supercenter on Des Moines's south side. He had, in his words, "manipulated my way out of a hospital in three days."

Zac texted Ali: "Hi, keep it a secret from everyone else please but they just released me from the looney bin lol I'm sorry for everything I had a like really bad episode Friday like all day"

Ali was worried sick. She'd known Zac had been in the psychiatric unit, but he hadn't called her; the phone was a community line, and he was embarrassed to call his girlfriend in front of other patients. His mom was on edge, too. Brenda is a fixer, the type of person who exhausts herself to make life easier for the people around her. Growing up as the fourth out of five children, she was always the peacemaker, the one trying to make things right. Now, as a mother, she'd been trying to save her middle son for months. Days before, she'd nearly lost him.

As his mom was paying the bill, Zac texted Ali again: "sorry if your embarrassed by me. I'm sure a lot of ppl are"

Ali: "Zachary joseph in no way am I embarrassed by you. Never would be."

Texts and calls came from friends and family. It seemed like people didn't quite know what to say. His old roommate Jake Powers texted him that night: "Hey bud, heard ya got got come home today! Just wanted to check in with you, and make sure you knew we were all thinking about ya this past week." Zac apologized: "I gues I'm literally losing my shit mental lol." He joked about it. He told Jake about his roommate in the psychiatric unit, there because he was a sex addict. Zac promised everyone he'd hit bottom and was on the road to recovery. The day after he was released from the inpatient psychiatric unit, he was scheduled to come back for a psychiatric evaluation.

But deep down, Zac wasn't so confident he could fix his damaged brain or the accompanying addictions. "The sober life sucks lol," he texted Ali. He told her about the night terrors that he'd been experiencing, searing dreams that woke him up in a choking fear and that made a good night's sleep impossible. He was always tired but could never sleep. During waking hours, his mind skittered like a dragonfly, a hundred things a minute. But the primary emotion was shame—shame that the big, strong Zac Easter, football captain and army badass, inheritor of the Easter Mentality, was now the talk of the town after his darkest, weakest moment. "If you could kind of keep it on the down low," he texted Jake, "I appreciate that."

Text exchange between Zac and Ali, Tuesday, November 17, 2015:

ZAC: I got to tell you truth I've kind of been holding back on, I feel highly emotional unstable right now lol
ALI: Can you try to explain in what ways you feel emotionally unstable . . .
ZAC: idk my emotions are truly just fucked and all over the place. One minute I'm all happy and the next minute I just feel hopeless on life
ALI: Can I call ya
ZAC: it might be easier for me to txt for a min
ALI: We can text then! When you say you feel hopeless do you know why you feel hopeless or is it more of an unexplainable feeling of hopelessness—like you don't know why you feel that way?

ZAC: Yeah idk why. It's miserable lol. Actually sometimes it's both

ALI: Sometimes it's both what

ZAC: Sometimes I know why I feel that way and sometimes I don't

ALI: Well when you know why, what's the reason

ZAC: Just all my shit is not going to get better and I feel like I just lie to people and say yay I'm going to get better, but in reality it's really a long shit in hell

ALI: Why don't you think you'll get better

ZAC: Let's be honest lol. You can't fix a brain

Text exchange between Zac and Ali, the morning of Saturday, November 21, 2015:

ZAC: Aren't you a little mad or embarrassed by my actions?

ALI: I am in no way embarrassed or mad by last week. I was only extremely worried and upset and anxious until I got to talk to you. Please believe me when I say in no way was/am I mad at you or embarrassed.

ZAC: I know but I feel bad because I totally about committed suicide and went to the loony bin lol

ALI: Zac in that moment you weren't you and you had a lot eating away at you because you haven't felt like you were in control of your life . . . but you shouldn't feel bad. What's important is that you're still here and that you're getting help. If I was mad or embarrassed I would've left by now— clearly that hasn't happened :p

ZAC: Yeah I'm still not feeling to well overall ;(

ALI: It definitely takes time babe and that's why I think it's

really good to go to a therapist once a week for awhile. Do
you wanna try to explain what/how you're feeling right now?
Zac: Not something you want to hear, but most day I wonder why I'm still alive . . . the hopelessness just gets to me
Ali: Well I think you're alive because there's a reason for
you to be. You're the incredible person who has so much
potential and so much ahead of you and you're alive because
of that. You're one of the strongest and most resilient people
I know because there's a reason you're supposed to be here
and be alive . . . even if you can't see that some days.
Zac: I won't lie, and I'd like to get this off my chest. Some
days I almost think it would be best for you if you didn't
have a guy like me. Like yes I know I'm a good guy in general, but I do carry a lot of baggage and I just don't want
to hurt you by doing some actions I feel like I can't always
control. Like last Friday, that was my 4th suicide attempt . . .
like clearly something is fucked up in me . . . I feel like I'm
sliding down my mountain and I'm doing all I can to try and
to go back up
Ali: I get what you're saying, but what is best for me is for
you to get better. And I don't care about how much baggage
you have—I love you and want to be with you and there
for you and want to help you get better in any way I can.
Your baggage isn't scaring me away. But I'm not just blowing smoke up your ass when I say you can get better . . . I
truly believe theres a reason youre still here and that as hard
as things are now, they will get better and you will get past
this and achieve all the amazing things you have ahead of
you . . . especially now that you're not doing it or dealing
with this on your own anymore.

Zac: Your best babe! Your truly a special person that I don't even understand yet, I mean that in a good way ;) But yeah your right. I'll get it figured and now I have more of a support system! Especially you :)

Text exchange between Zac and Ali, Tuesday, November 24, 2015, before Ali returned to Iowa for Thanksgiving break:

Zac: Omg I did this to myself but I can't go [to therapy] today lol

Ali: Yes you can babe. It'll be okay. The hardest part is getting up and going but this could be really beneficial for you and help you get the ball rolling on getting past all of this. And I'm here to talk whenever you need me today. And just try stay calm. Remember why you're going to get better and healthier—and just keep looking forward to seeing me :) Baby steps

Zac: Lol I know babe! Your the bestest

Ali: Text me whenever you have a break and tell me how its going. It's all about attitude, remember? Just stay open to letting it help you!!

Zac, a bit later: Yeah fuxk I can't do it

Ali: Did you go for any of it?

Zac: no just sat in the parking lot

Thanksgiving 2015: A chilly, rainy, windy day in the cornfields surrounding the Easter household. As the family gorged themselves on traditional Thanksgiving fixings, the skies turned to a nasty wintry mix of rain, snow, and freezing rain. That did not discourage

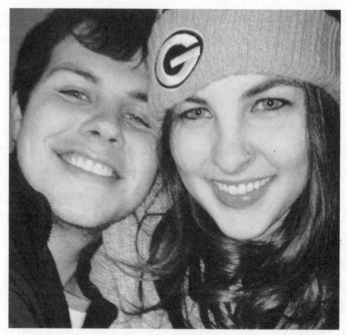

*Zac turned Ali into a football fan, and they
watched his Green Bay Packers together.*

most of the Easter family from heading to early-bird Black Friday
sales on Thanksgiving night.

Alone in the Easter basement, Zac and Ali burrowed into the
ratty old couch. They cradled plates of leftover Thanksgiving food
and tuned the television to NBC. Zac was excited for another of
America's favorite Thanksgiving traditions: football. Zac's beloved
Green Bay Packers were taking on their archrival, the Chicago
Bears, at the wet, wind-whipped Lambeau Field in Wisconsin. The
game was certainly important for football reasons: The Packers
and Vikings were tied atop the NFC North after the Packers had
just gone to Minneapolis and won a road game. The Bears were
4–6 and desperate for a win. Zac shouted at the television in glee

in the first quarter when Packers quarterback Aaron Rodgers hit running back Eddie Lacy for a twenty-five-yard touchdown pass for the first points of the game. But this game was important for nostalgic reasons, too, and as it entered halftime—traditionally when the eighty thousand fans at Lambeau Field flee to bathrooms and concession stands—fans instead remained in their seats. Zac stared at the television as the cameras focused in on his favorite football player of all time. That player waited nervously in the stadium tunnel for the ceremony to retire his number, the giant yellow 4 forever hanging above the box seats in Lambeau Field's north end zone.

Brett Favre had played sixteen seasons for the Packers, winning one Super Bowl and three NFL MVP awards as one of the top quarterbacks of his generation. But Favre's legend was based more on his attitude, the swashbuckling, devil-may-care way he approached the game of football. He played through pain and injuries. He started an NFL-record 321 consecutive games. He didn't miss a single game from 1992 until 2010. During that period, though, the sport took its toll. In 1996, Favre suffered a seizure during a hospital visit. It was later revealed that he had developed an addiction to the opioid Vicodin to cope with the daily pain of being an NFL warrior. He went to in-patient treatment for forty-six days in the off-season. Yet he never missed a game.

As his Hall of Fame career continued, Favre kept battling through injuries—some of them quite serious. There was one summer when he didn't remember a single one of his daughter's soccer games that he attended. His consecutive game streak came to an end in December 2010, when he missed a game due to a sprained shoulder. One week later, though, Favre was back on the field, and he sustained a concussion while playing for the Minnesota Vikings.

A Chicago Bears player had sacked Favre. He was knocked out for at least ten seconds. As Favre lay on the field, the Vikings trainer shook him. The trainer heard him snoring. Then, Favre came to. Woozy, he was helped to his feet by the trainer. The legendary quarterback looked at the trainer and said, "What are the Bears doing here?" That marked Favre's final appearance in an NFL game.

Now, though, Zac watched as the crowd gave him a hero's welcome. As the public-address announcer lauded Favre as a "possessor of legendary durability," the camera captured the legend, the hood of his raincoat obscuring part of his face. He looked unnerved. His eyes darted back and forth. "At quarterback," the announcer said, "from Southern Mississippi . . . number four . . . BRETT FAVRE!"

The crowd cheered. Zac turned to Ali. He recognized in Favre the same tics he'd experienced himself. "I wouldn't be surprised if he has CTE," Zac told her. "He looks so anxious right now. And his face is all red."

At midfield, Favre stepped out from under his umbrella, and the Packers' president passed the microphone to him. Of course, Favre first gave an homage to toughness. "This is Green Bay weather!" Favre said, as winds slapped against thousands of yellow number-4 flags fans held in the air. "I love it. I love it."

Zac had been struggling with being in front of people, had become terrified of public speaking, which he blamed on the concussions. "I can just tell that's what he's feeling, too," Zac told Ali.

In 2018, Favre opened up to journalist Megyn Kelly on NBC. He told her he suffered "probably thousands" of concussions during his playing career. He said that he learned at a young age from his football coach father that you should never come out of a practice or game just because of "a little head ding." You didn't want to be called a "sissy." Yet at age forty-seven, Favre now said his short-term memory was already failing him, and that coming up with the right words in conversation was becoming difficult. He worried that he might be experiencing the early symptoms of CTE.

"No matter what I do to try to take care of myself physically, that is a part of my future that I really can't control," Favre told Kelly. "And that is very scary."

He told Kelly he'd prefer that his grandchildren played golf, not football. Around the time of that year's Super Bowl, Favre appeared on CNN to speak with journalist Christiane Amanpour about head injuries. "Tomorrow I may not remember who I am, I may not know where I live—and that's the frightening thing for us football players," he told Amanpour.

"How does one make the game safer?" she asked Favre.

"How do you make the game safer?" he replied. "You don't play."

ZAC'S MOODS WEREN'T just ping-ponging. They were rocketing back and forth. One minute, he was pledging to go to all his therapy appointments and conquer all his demons. He was going to be the old Zac again. The next minute, he was filled with self-loathing. It was after midnight when Ali left his parents' house. Their Saturday night had turned into a Sunday morning on November 29, 2015. In a few hours, she would head back to law school for her final couple of weeks of the semester. At 1:55 a.m., Zac texted her, his words filled with gratitude: "Thanks for being my Winslow, I'll never be able to say it enough. P.s please please watch for deer!" Then, he went to sleep. But two hours later, he was up, bulldozed awake by another bad dream. Instead of trying to go back to sleep,

Zac walked outside and opened the trunk of Big Red, where he had stashed a bottle of liquor. He took it to his room and started drinking. He sent Ali a drunken, rambling, 356-word text shortly before sunrise. It read in part: "I guess one thing that's holding me back from [trying to get better] is to still being kind of on the edge of just wanting to die, and just say fuxk trying to get better because I'm tired of it . . . thanks for saving my life that night, I know you may not want to hear it but if you wouldn't of called id be a goner . . . I love you so much it's stupid!"

The next morning, Zac went for a walk in the woods. His mother peeked in his room and found the empty liquor bottle. She confronted him about it and gave him a lecture: He'd never fix his brain unless he stopped drinking. And she'd found something else, too, while searching online: an inpatient clinic in California that specialized in people with brain injuries and chemical dependency issues. She pushed him to try it. Zac didn't want to. His dad joined the discussion, too.

When his parents finished lecturing him, Zac texted Ali: "I'm so sorry Winslow. Idk what happened to me last night ;(. . . I'm a fuck up ;("

The next day, a Monday, Zac went to his first Alcoholics Anonymous meeting.

He told Ali that he was feeling delusional, that the world was trying to manipulate him.

At 6:15 a.m. on Tuesday, December 1, 2015, Ali texted Zac: "Baby are you ok"

"Oh lord no," Zac replied. "I woke up and had a minor freak out. I drank again . . .

"I'm worthless"

Text exchange between Zac and Ali on Friday, December 4, 2015:

ALI: I'm sorry you're having an off day

ZAC: I know, sorry you have to deal with it. It's not fair to you

ALI: Nothing unfair babe. And nothing I have to 'deal with.' You're my boyfriend and I love you - just our current situation and you're just dealing with stuff that I'm helping you through. I choose to and want to

ZAC: Thanks babe. Please run though whenever I get to bad. You deserve better ;)

ALI: I deserve what I choose and I choose you. And you deserve all the best just the same. I'm never gonna run - already told you you can't get rid of me. And no more getting bad babe—this is a turning point in your life and you're gonna get better.

ZAC: You have a lovely brain ;)

ALI: You do, too.

ALI: Also, i know you don't want to talk about it but I just want to say that I really think you should go to treatment tomorrow/this week and definitely therapy and i hope that you do. Not just because we have a headbutt [their phrase for a pinkie swear] on it but also because you can't do this on your own and you shouldn't have to and if you let it, those things will help you get better.

Zac apologized. He apologized for his mood swings, he apologized for skipping therapy, he apologized for feeling hopeless and just wanting to drink away the pain.

ZAC: Idk I'm just a fucked up soul . . . I'm hopeless sometimes, I'm hopeful sometimes, and then there's when I'm
happy just drinking and jamming to music. I've been
depressed for so long idk what feeling in a normal mood
means. I'm sorry but honestly you are beating a dead horse
and that's me, I'm just scared shitless and my emotions
are all over the place. You deserve better than me, I wish
I wasn't that guy. I know we're in love and we mean it.
It's just hard and I'm scared I'm wearing both of us down
sometimes. But one thing I do know is that I'll make it like
I always have. You may seem annoyed and I get that. But
I will always come around because I always do. I guess
I'm waiting for myself to catch on to that mindset and
fight through it. With the mindset I have now, idk if I can
make it.

ALI: You're not weighing us both down and you and I are
fine. I know you're scared. I know that's what is holding
you back, but that's also why you need treatment (and
most importantly, to see your therapist weekly)—to help
make you realize that being sober isn't scary and will
actually help you feel happiness and love and excitement
ten times stronger because it'll no longer be clouded by
substances . . . You're not a fucked up soul. And you're not
hopeless.

ZAC: I know you and my family love me and it keeps me
going, but some days shit is just messed up in my head.
Another reason I'm scared of being sober is because when
I'm sober I can't feel anything. I could cut myself sober and
not feel a thing. I'm not a cutter by any means and I have
done it once before to just check myself, but just saying. The

numbness I feel sober is what kills me inside. I need to figure out how not to be numb sober. I know that and therapy will help. It's just exhausting even thinking about it. That's why I didn't want to talk about it earlier. Substances help me feel and that's not okay . . . When I'm with you I don't feel so numb.

ALI: I know you're fighting babe, I'm just trying to help and don't want you to do it alone or feel alone.

ZAC: I guess I'm just mentally sick and there's no certain medicine for it. I wish I could pick you up on a private jet and chain you to the wall like 50 shades. I'm tired of this like I promise and it's either sink or swim. And I WaNT to learn how to swim lol.

ZAC'S DAD TOOK all the guns out of the house, packing them in a big toolbox and stashing them at his brother's house. They took all the alcohol out of the house. Everyone in the family was constantly on edge. There came to be a morbid rhythm to Zac's daily successes and failures: He went to Alcoholics Anonymous meetings, but then he'd wake up in the middle of the night and start drinking.

Something had shifted inside him. No longer did he worry that he might be going crazy; now, he was *certain* of it. Fatalism swept over him. He told his mother he'd made a bucket list: "Things to Do Before CTE Takes Away My Mind." Travel overseas. Camp in the timber in winter. Go rattlesnake hunting on the family's land. "I think I'm going to hike across the country because I only got so much time before I lose my mind," he told his mom.

On December 5, 2015, the sixth anniversary of the day Zac bagged his ten-point buck, Myles Sr. decided to take his son hunting. Perhaps they could recapture some of the tranquility of the old days. They got up before sunrise, ate bacon and eggs, and got in the truck by 5:15 a.m.

The forty-minute drive from their house to the family's timber was a good time to talk. They sipped coffee. Myles told his son that he was proud of him, that Zac was smart and talented and successful. He said they would fight through this as a family. "I'm sorry about the concussions from football," he told his son. "I didn't understand it earlier." Zac didn't want his dad feeling guilty. He told him that he loved football. He told him he even missed football. He didn't tell his father that he was losing hope that he would get better—giving voice to something like that was incompatible with the Easter mentality—but he did tell his father that he often heard voices in his head. Later, Myles would wish he'd asked his son what the voices were telling him. Instead, uncomfortable to dig deeper into his son's mental struggles, he ignored the comment.

They got out of the truck. Zac watched his dad remove the shotguns from behind the seat, where he'd stashed them after picking them up from Zac's uncle a couple of nights before the hunt. Myles handed his son a shotgun. "You're not going to shoot yourself, right?" he said. Zac laughed: "Not in front of you." They both laughed. "OK, I knew you wouldn't," Myles said. Zac's older brother met them, and together the three Easter men hiked into the woods. They didn't see a deer that day, but it didn't matter. From the tree stand Myles Sr. was heartened by the sight of two of his boys walking down the hill together, laughing. In that moment, at least, Zac seemed like his old self. "I thought maybe we were getting better," Myles Sr. recalled later. But his older son saw something that worried him. "When we were walking in the dark," Myles II told his father, "I turned around and looked at him and he was talking to himself. His lips were moving."

They hunted till after sunset. On the ride home, Myles Sr. picked up a six-pack of Coors Light tallboys for them to split. Zac's mom wouldn't have liked this—alcohol, she knew, only made his problems worse—but, hell, Myles just wanted to go back to the way things used to be. It was only a couple of beers. As they rumbled home along the gravel country roads, beers in hand, Zac turned to his father. "This was one of the best days I've had," he said.

Zac and his dad fell asleep next to each other in the living room, watching Iowa play Michigan State in the Big Ten championship game. It was a tough, ugly defensive battle, the exact kind of football game they loved.

A COUPLE OF days later, Brenda Easter came home to find Zac's car gone from the driveway. This was odd. Brenda had been keeping track of his every move, and he was usually at home. He did not answer his phone when she called. She called Ali; Ali called Zac again and again. He didn't pick up.

She texted him: "Baby what's going on—your mom said you took off?"

And then: "Where are you babe?"

Ali started freaking out. Brenda started freaking out. It felt like the events of Friday the 13th all over again. Zac had told plenty of people that he just wanted to disappear for a while to clear his head. No one took him seriously. Best-case scenario, Ali thought, was that he'd just gone for a walk in the woods to prove people wrong.

Ali texted him again: "Zac please tell me you're okay and call me."

Finally, Zac responded: "I'm ok and I'm in Oklahoma;)"

He told Ali he'd been feeling cooped up at his parents' house, sitting there thinking about losing his mind, and he needed to get away. So a few hours earlier he'd emptied his parents' cabinets of food, gotten in his car, and just started driving. He was heading for Oklahoma, but then he turned around and started making his way back; after a wrong turn, he wound up in Kansas City and got a hotel room for the night. Zac ordered pizza and stayed in his hotel room. Then, he went to a strip club.

The next morning, he turned around and drove home.

Email from Zac to Ali, later in the day after Zac drove back from Kansas City:

From: Zachary Easter <zeaster1@hotmail.com>
Date: Tue, Dec 8, 2015 at 2:36 PM
Subject: i love you
To: Alison Epperson <xxxx@gmail.com>

Dear Winslow,
First off, I just want to thank You for being You! You have an amazing heart and I'm so blessed to have someone like you in my life. I love you so much I can't even come up with some of those cheesy saying talking about how "Words can't describe how much I love you" type of stuff, so I'm just going to keep it real and original ☺ Your the rock that keeps me my sole from blowing in the wind. (Cheesy I know, but so is macaroni and cheese and I know how much you love that lol) Since some things have changed since the last time I wrote this I guess I'm glad I got a chance to update some things.

Your law professors won't appreciate my grammar in this letter, but they can get bent for giving you so much work lol.

Looking back over the years I can't help but laugh and smile about our story. If our story was a song we'd kick Taylor Swifts ass on the top charts lol. I remember our first sober moments together being flirty with each other on the senior bench and who would of known then what the two of us would have grown into. From the barn in literally negative temperatures to the sun shining on us at Grey's Lake we've come a long way together and I will never for one second regret any of it. I will admit I do kind of regret not telling about my feelings for you sooner, but screw it! It must have been meant for us to turn out this way and it only makes our song even better with the fact that I told you I first loved you when I was puking my guts out that one night while you held my hair back haha ☺

I wish you the best of luck on all your exams babe! You've come so fare this year I could never be more proud of you!!! You've been working your ass off school and trying to balance all that stuff while trying to balance a relationship with a guy like me is something I wish upon no one lol! You're the only one I know with enough resilience to deal with my shit ☺. For that, may god bless you haha! I think your sleeping now, but I can't wait until we cuddle naked and just takes naps with your hair in my face. Moments like that are the ones I live for. Well that's about a page and just what's on my mind for now. Definitely not the traditional love letter, but I hope I found a way to spark a smile on your face somehow ☺

Oh and one more thing, p.s. I love you!

Zac

Text exchange between Zac and Ali, Wednesday, December 9, 2015:

ZAC: This is stupid

ALI: What is baby

ZAC: Idk this whole life I'm living

ALI: Don't say that baby. Things WILL get better. I know it's overwhelming and scary but you're gonna get through this and if you open yourself up to it this program can really help you. You have so much ahead of you baby and despite everything going on you're a great person and have great things in your life and treatment will make all of that better and more apparent and you'll be able to really feel and enjoy everything you've got going for you

ZAC: Yeah I guess

ALI: It's gonna be okay baby. Give yourself a little bit of time to think things over and decide when you wanna go and what you're gonna do in the meantime. I'm always gonna be here. I love you

ZAC: Love you to

ON THE AFTERNOON of Saturday, December 12, 2015, Ali was home for winter break. Zac texted her he was sick of his mom—"she's giving me some motivational speech"—and he was going to run away. "Fuck I just don't care anymore," Zac texted her. "I don't want to be get Better"

ALI: Do you want me to come pick you up and we can drive around and talk and clear your mind a little?

ZAC: If you help buy me a beer so I can calm my emotions before hand lol

ALI: Zac . . . why don't we try to calm your emotions without that first

ZAC: By doing what

ALI: Driving and talking and being with each other

ZAC: Sure

ALI: Okay. Almost to dealerships and coming straight to you

ZAC: No offense but that's not going to help me

ALI: Well alcohol isn't going to help in the long run either. It'll just make it worse. Only a quick fix. And it's better than sitting at home stewing in your emotions

ZAC: I'm craving a drink because that's the only way I know how to do it, so it's up to you. If I leave here I'm going to get a drink lol

ALI: Not if your with me. Why don't we try to deal with it without a drink together

ZAC: Because what is that going to do? No you might as well not come over. No offense I'm just going to talk you into leaving

ALI: And who says you're gonna be able to talk me into leaving uh? I'm just as stubborn and I'm already on my way

ZAC: God your stubborn lol

ALI: And you don't know any other way to deal because you've always gone to alcohol. You haven't tried much else. It's not gonna hurt to try zac. Fuck yeah I'm stubborn.

ZAC: I really don't think I want to talk to anyone right now truthfully

ALI: Well then don't talk. Just drive with me

ZAC: You can drive me to a gas station lol

ALI: Nahh. Don't need gas

ZAC: Then please don't come

ALI: Too bad. Too far to turn around. Sucks you gotta hang
with your girlfriend

ZAC: I'm not showered my breath stinks

ALI: I've got gum

ZAC: Your not helping

ZAC: I'm happy when I'm drinking by myself in my sweet
misery. I'm not happy doing anything else and all I do is
fake it

ALI: Then let me help. Sitting alone at home angry or drinking isn't helping either

ZAC: I'm a broken man and you should leave me!

ALI: And that's the problem. That's not healthy and that's
not real happiness. I'm on your street. Will you please come
out

ZAC: Come and do what? I'm in my room

Ali walked into the Easters' house. Brenda was sitting on the
couch, at a loss. Ali went upstairs and opened the door to Zac's
room. He was lying on his bed, staring at the ceiling. She snuggled
up next to him. He was quiet.

It was time for tough love. She didn't have many cards left to
play.

"Are you going to fucking talk to me?" she asked.

"*What?*" he said. "What do you want me to say?"

He didn't want to go to California to the rehabilitation clinic
his mother had researched. He didn't think it would work.

"What's the fucking point?" Zac told Ali. "What's the purpose
anymore? What am I doing here?"

Ali started crying.

"I'm a purpose, Zac," she said. "You say you love me. If you're
not going to do it for yourself, why won't you do it for me?"

Zac got quiet. Tears welled in his eyes.

She looked directly into his eyes.

"Am I not worth it?" she asked. "Can you try to stay alive for me?"

"I do love you," he said. "You are worth trying for. I want to try for you. I just don't know what's going to help at this point."

ZAC WAS SPENDING a lot of time alone in his bedroom. One night—Wednesday, December 16, 2015—he went downstairs. Myles Sr. was sitting on the couch.

"Hey, Dad," Zac said. "That thing on Mike Webster is on Channel 11." It was the two-hour PBS documentary, "League of Denial: The NFL's Concussion Crisis," a *Frontline* segment about concussions and the ties between football and long-term brain injuries. Zac sat at the top of the stairs, watching his dad watch the documentary. It was as if Zac felt his dad could understand more about his own struggles from watching the show. Once he was sure his dad would watch the whole thing, Zac went back into his bedroom and shut the door.

IT HAD BEEN a fun week with Ali home from law school. Slowly, Zac warmed to the idea of inpatient treatment in California. He told his family he would go right after Christmas. Zac and Ali cuddled in the Easters' basement and watched *Shameless*. They went on a date night at Okoboji Grill on Des Moines's south side and stopped at a drive-through frozen custard joint on the way home. They sat at the kitchen table and helped Zac's mom stuff envelopes for her job at the Indianola Chamber of Commerce. Nick Haworth, Zac's old buddy, came by one night, and he joined Zac and Ali at McDonald's, then watched the Mark Wahlberg comedy *Ted 2* with them. There were times when Zac felt anxious, but on the whole, Ali thought he'd turned a corner. All week, they had good sex—great sex, even, the type of sex where there are only two people in the world who exist. Zac told her that when they had sex, that was one of the few times when he never doubted his connection to humanity. There were so many things in Zac's life he felt disconnected from, sometimes to the point where he couldn't tell what was real and what was not. Sex with Ali was an emotional connection that he knew was real, without a doubt.

On Friday, December 18, they planned to spend the whole day together. Ali's sisters were due back home that night, so it would be the only day when they had Ali's parents' house to themselves. Ali picked him up in the morning. He felt terrible—stomachache, headache—but they went to her parents' house anyway. They sat on the big blue recliner together and watched *Shameless*. They ordered pizza and french fries from Winn's Pizza & Steakhouse, and they drove to the town square to pick up their food. Zac helped Ali get the artificial Christmas tree out of the garage and set it up. Later that night, Zac was going to take Ali out to dinner, just the two of them, and stop by to say hi to her parents beforehand. But first, he needed a nap and a haircut, so Ali drove him home. In the car, they listened to their song, "Technicolor Beat," by a band called Oh Wonder, a song about true love helping a person conquer his biggest fears.

They held hands. "I know I didn't feel well today," Zac told Ali as she drove, "but I want you to know I had an amazing day today. I loved today. It was like a perfect day. I was so happy to just be there with you." She pulled into his parents' driveway. He got out, came by the driver's side, put his head in her window, and gave her a kiss: "I love you."

It was after 7:00 p.m. when Zac left the house to get his hair cut. The Easters had family pictures scheduled for the next day.

When he got home after 8:00 p.m., his mom was asleep in bed with the television on, sick with a headache. Zac's dad was upstairs, trying to give Tito, their fat, white Rat Terrier, a bath. He had taken the dogs hunting out back. Tito found a possum and killed it, but not without a fight. The dog was covered in blood.

"You're in deep shit if mom sees that," Zac told his dad as he walked into the bathroom with Tito.

"Can you help me out here?" Myles said. Then, he looked up at his son. "You got your hair cut," he said admiringly. "Boy, you sure look good."

Zac helped his dad wrestle the dog into the tub. Soon, the bath-water ran red. Then, Zac disappeared into his room.

He canceled dinner with Ali. She asked if he wanted to come out later, when she was heading to downtown Des Moines with friends. No thanks, he said. He still wasn't feeling well, not mentally and not physically, so he was just going to stay at home.

Ever since the suicide attempt, Myles and Brenda had been watching Zac like hawks. Their scrutiny was part of why he was so annoyed with his parents; he felt like he'd lost his independence. Myles planted himself on the couch at the bottom of the stairs, to make sure his son couldn't get past undetected.

But soon, Myles drifted off to sleep.

From his room, Zac texted with Ali.

ZAC: Ha that was pretty fun [day] with you ;) , . . I apologize things are different now

ALI: Things may be a little different but we are still us and still love each other and still have great moments every time we are together. Don't apologize

ZAC: You say don't apologize but I really need to. God only knows how much you've been through it all with for the downtimes and the best nights of our lives. I'm sorry for my the emotional toll it's had to have taken on you some-nights.

ALI: I willingly take it all on because I love you. I appreciate that you recognize I'm in this too but just keep loving me and being open to getting help and working on things and letting me in and I'll be okay.

ZAC: I know babe. I've said it before, but your a beautiful person with a beautiful [heart] who sees the good in others. My struggles just keep overwhelming me and I hate how it comes off to you ;(

Ali was at a table at Johnny's Hall of Fame, a sports bar in downtown Des Moines, with a group of friends. Jake Powers, Zac's old roommate, noticed she was quiet and distracted, looking at her phone. He asked if anything was wrong. She told him Zac was having a bad day. She went to the bar's atrium to text with him privately.

At the Easters' house, Zac opened the door of his room and crept down the stairs. He grabbed his father's car keys off the coffee table, passing within inches of his dad. For years afterward, Myles would wonder what was going through Zac's mind as he walked past. Zac went to the basement, opened a box filled with shotgun slugs, and took one. He opened the door to his dad's truck, slid behind the seats, and pulled out the 20-gauge shotgun his dad had got him for his birthday more than a decade before.

In downtown Des Moines, Ali moved with the group to a country music bar called Beer Can Alley. She kept texting with Zac.

ALI: You've always been one of the few people I hold on a pedestal and think the most about. And that's cuz your a great person and a beautiful and special soul. I'll never think differently and you'll be deep in my heart forever because of it. I know that's super cheesy and sappy but completely true all the same.

ZAC: Thanks, babe. I really needed that. I'm kind of down tonight

ALI: I know you are. But know there's a light at the end of the tunnel and a huge fucking bright light for you . . . I'll always believe in you even on your worst days. Takes time and lots of effort but you're the best and strongest person I know and you're gonna make it because on the days that you're the most hopeless I'll be there to lean on and remind you of the amazing things and people in your life and why you should have faith

ZAC: Your sole is beautiful. I won't lie, I've asked myself why a girl like you stays with a guy like me.

ALI: You've been the biggest constant in my life. I've never not had feelings for you and I believe that means something. I truly believe we were meant to be and no matter what happens with our relationship in the future (although I hope for only amazing things lol) I'll love you forever and always believe in you and always be there for you and never let you fall. I've never loved someone the way I love you and I'll never let that go.

ZAC: I know my feelings for you are real when I can't tell when every other feeling is real or fake. I may be slowly loosing my mind and I can't help that, but I do know your always going to be my Winslow ;)

ALI: You'll never really lose your mind with me around. I won't let you. I really really love you. And like you said, even [on] your worst days I know you truly love me. That feeling will always be real. Ps Jacob wants me to tell you high

ALI: Hi*

ZAC: Lol you got high and hi mixed up ;) is someone a little stoned? Lol and tell him I said hi back. And also tell him go pack go ;)

ALI: No I'm just typing fast . . .

ZAC: I love Alison for Alison

ALI: I love zac for zac

ZAC: I miss the old Zac. He was a nice guy with a loving heart. Idk who I am now

ALI: You're still a nice guy with a loving heart. I know you don't see that right now but I FEEL it every day. With time and work and help and medicine you'll feel yourself again. I 100% know this

ZAC: No thank you for everything. You've helped me through so much and never ever blame yourself for anything. I love you and will always be over your shoulder looking after you no matter what. Always keep having fun. Always remember me. Always keep striving for greatness or shall I say first female president. Never quit fighting for what you believe for ;) I love you Winslow.

ALI: I love you, too babe but that sounds so past tense and is making me worried. I don't want you to talk that way . . . Are you okay. Please be honest. I can call you

Zac didn't reply. Ali called. Her call went to voicemail after one ring. Sometimes he just fell asleep, and Ali didn't want to worry anybody by freaking out. But something felt off. She called again. No answer.

Ali texted him: "Seriously zac. I'm worried now. I know you're having an off day but it will be okay—I know you have the fight in you. Please talk to me"

Jake noticed the concern on Ali's face. "You want a beer?" he offered. She immediately started bawling. It was midnight. It dawned on Jake what could be happening. He grabbed Ali and their friends, walked out of the bar with them, and went straight to his pickup. They sped back to Indianola. Ali called Zac's older brother, Myles II, who called Brenda. "Hey, is Zac upstairs?" Myles II asked his sleeping mother. Zac's dad sprinted up the stairs to his middle son's room. Zac wasn't there. A note was on his bed, scrawled on a torn-out piece of white notebook paper. Myles grabbed his reading glasses and read the note, written in Zac's angular, messy script.

> *Please! Look on my computer and print off my story and last wishes to everyone. PLEASE FULLFILL MY last wishes!*
>
> *Make sure Ali gets her letters. I love her and watch over her.*
>
> *Also give my story to the rest of family, print off. Also post all of it on Facebook eventually.*
>
> *Dad I'm sorry I broke into your truck.*
>
> *Thank you all for wanting to help.*
>
> *But I can't be helped.*
>
> *Love Zac*

Myles frantically called his son. Zac didn't pick up. Zac's mom called Ali in a panic. She told Ali that Zac had left a note. Ali was crying hysterically in the back of Jake's truck. They all figured there was only one place Zac could have gone: Lake Ahquabi. They called the police.

Ali texted Zac: "Baby. It's winslow. Please think of me please talk to me. I believe in you. I know you're upset but please talk to me."

Nothing.

"I need you to text me back," Ali texted.

Brenda and Myles drove down the winding, tree-lined hill that led to the lake. A patrol car was already there. "I'm sorry," the police officer told them.

Zac's body was lying on the ground, a 20-gauge shotgun slug torn through his chest.

As Jake was pulling into the state park, an ambulance was leaving with its lights off. Ali bolted from the truck and vomited.

TEN

The Future

ZAC HAD PRINTED the thirty-nine-page, double-spaced Microsoft Word document and left it in his room, by his desk, before he went to the basement to retrieve the shotgun slug. Titled "Concussions: My Silent Struggle," it was a brief autobiography of how those football concussions had led him to this. (His handwritten journals were stashed nearby in a file box.) After getting his story down, he went back to the beginning of the document and inserted a pre-amble of sorts.

> My last wishes
>
> IT's taken me about 5 months to write all of this. Sorry for the bad grammar in a lot of spots.
>
> I WANT MY BRAIN DONATED TO THE BRAIN BANK!! I WANT MY BRAIN DONATED TO THE SPORTS LEGACY INSTITUE A.K.A THE CONCUSSION FOUNDATION. If you go to the concussion foundation website you can see where there is a spot for donatation. I want my brain donated because I don't know what happened to me and I know the concussions had something to do with it.
>
> Please please please give me the cheapest burial possible. I don't want anything fancy and I want to be cremated. Once

cremated, I want my ashes spread in the timber on the side hill where I shot my 10 point buck. That is where I was happiest and that I where I want to lay. Feel free to spread my ashes around the timber if you'd like, but just remember on the side hill is where I would like most of my remains. I am truly sorry if I put you in a financial burden. I just cant live with this pain any more.

I don't want anything expensive at my funeral or what ever it is. Please please please I beg you to chose the cheapest route and not even buy me a burial plot at a cemetary. It is what I, Zac Easter WANTS!!

I also do not want a military funeral If there are color guardsmen or anyone else at my funerial or whatever you have I will haunt you forever. I DO NOT WANT A MILITARY FUNERIAL. I DON'T WANT THE MILITATRY ENVOVLED AT ALL. Fuck the army and fuck the government . . .

You will have to turn in my military equipment in though. That is in the trunk of my car in a green army duffle bag and stuff in levi's room like my uniforms . . . Please tell them my story.

Levi gets my car, it will need a oil change and breaks/tires done her shortly. Please take care of old red. It will need cleaned out as well because I am a slob.

Thank you for being the best family in the world. I will watch over you all and please take my last wishes into consideration. Do not do something I do no want. Just remember, I don't want a military funeral like grandpas. It is my last wishes and last rights.

I am with the lord now.

- Look, Im sorry every one for the choice I made. Its wrong and we all know it.

FAMILY AND FRIENDS gathered at the Easter household that night. They stayed almost until sunrise. They cried. They hugged. Zac's older brother punched a hole in a wall.

For much of the next forty-eight hours, Zac's dad stood outside in the cold. He didn't want to talk to anyone. Regret was almost suffocating him. Myles Easter would pick up his son's autobiography once, shortly after his death. He read through the entire thing, just one time, trying to understand what had happened to his son's tortured mind. Standing out in the cold, he was numb. As family and friends gathered in the Easters' home to share in their grief, not many came up to talk with him. "Nobody," Myles Sr. recalled later, "knew what the hell to say."

FOUR DAYS LATER, Eric Kluver, the head football coach at Indianola High School, stood over his former player's casket. Inside was the body of the young man who represented everything Kluver loved about football, the wild child who for two summers put in some good, honest work alongside him in the sweltering Iowa heat. Later, Kluver would pin photographs from Zac's funeral to the walls of his basement. He didn't want to forget any of this, or the feeling of guilt that maybe he had helped create this moment.

Did football do this? he thought as he stood over the casket. *Did I do this?* He and his staff had always taught Zac proper tackling technique, of course, but they'd never insisted that he scale back his aggression. If anything, that aggression—the feeling that Zac would sacrifice his own body for the good of the team—made him an easy role model for younger players. Zac's body might not have been the ideal football body, but his mentality—his mind—was the archetype: the hard-nosed player every football coach dreams of.

And yet his story became the superhero movie that ends in tragedy: Zac Easter's greatest strength turned out to be his greatest weakness.

Kluver knew football played a role in Zac's destruction: football, and the culture around America's favorite sport. He could compartmentalize the life-altering injuries to Matt Hanke and Joey Goodale as freak brain injuries that happened to occur on a football field. But Zac? This was from *football*, and from the way Zac played the sport for nearly half his life, since when he was a little kid until he graduated from high school. It was like the old dilemma from football's earliest days: unnecessary roughness versus necessary roughness. The violence that's outside the bounds of the game's propriety versus the violence that this game glorifies. Zac's injury felt like, quite simply, part of the game, at least the old-fashioned, hard-hitting, devil-may-care way that Zac played the game.

"To see him lying in that casket," Kluver said later, "you would think that would be enough to make you say that enough is enough. It almost makes me sick to keep doing what I'm doing."

And yet, months after saying this, Kluver would lead his high school football team out of the sparkling new locker room at Indianola High School for its first game of the new season. In the hallways of the school, he would still see the occasional BIG HAMMER T-shirt worn by a younger brother of a player who had earned one many years ago, before Kluver stopped handing them out to reward the most bone-crunching of hits.

Despite everything, Kluver still believes in football. He believes more good comes from the sport than bad. Far more good. He

believes life is full of risks, and that we should not pad our children in Bubble Wrap. Boys must be boys. But his faith in football
is rattled. When I told him Zac wrote in parts of his journal that
he wished he'd never played football, Kluver squeezed his eyes shut
and put a hand to his forehead.

"There's definitely been times where I've said, 'Is this worth it?'"
the coach said.

What Kluver was debating inside his own mind parallels perhaps the defining question of this era in American sports: Is football worth it? Or, to put a finer point on it: What are we willing
to sacrifice as a society to keep our beloved national sport recognizable as the same sport we have enjoyed—the sport that has
helped shape us as a country—for more than a century? If 10
percent of NFL players end up with shortened lives and with less
quality of life due to brain injuries sustained by playing the sport,
is that an acceptably low number for us to continue as unabated,
unabashed fans of the sport? What if that number is 25 percent?
Or 50 percent? (The best guesses of current science indicate former NFL players die with brain disease at much higher rates,
somewhere between 5 and 8 percent, than the normal population.)
And how does that determination change when we are talking
about collegiate players, who are paid not in the millions of dollars but in scholarships that cover tuition and room and board?
It is one thing when old football warriors suffer from bad knees
and constant joint pain. Every football player since the sport's
beginning has known these pains later in life were the price of
admission. But the idea that this sport could severely damage
the brain, the ability to reason—the very thing that makes us
human—changes the equation into something closer to an existential crisis.

Another more complicated part of the equation: What about the Zac Easters of our world? What level of risk are we willing to take on as a society when we are talking about the ways that football hurts the high school standouts who'll never advance to the highest levels of this sport? For a teenager with zero shot at the pros—someone who goes into sports for the fun and the camaraderie and maybe even the life lessons—is playing on a football team a significantly better life experience than playing a sport with a lower chance of permanent brain trauma: basketball or baseball or track? Bennet Omalu, the neuropathologist who helped bring CTE to the public consciousness, zeroes in on this point. He's become a controversial figure in scientific circles for many reasons, not the least of which is that his research has segued into what often feels like a campaign against youth playing contact sports. He does not blame the NFL for the current concussion crisis. But his solution for how society should wrestle with this is as simple and practical as it is threatening to football's existence, and he argues it with an evangelical fervor.

Here's what Omalu argues: He compares football to smoking. Both are dangerous, and both are things that some humans enjoy. So make tackle football like smoking: something that American men are only permitted to do after they turn eighteen. This approach would protect the Zac Easters of the world from any sort of brain trauma related to youth or high school football, and would also limit the years that a college or professional football player is exposed to repetitive hits to the head. But this solution likely would also dry out the talent pool for college football and the NFL. I think it's fair to assume a ban on tackle football for youths younger than eighteen would within a couple of generations cause the marginalization, or even extinction, of college and professional football.

"What Zac's case tells us is that parents need to know that when you put a helmet on your son's head and send him out to play football, there is a risk of your child suffering permanent brain damage," Omalu told me. "The truth is inconvenient. The truth could be painful. This is a game people love. But as a society we evolve. And as we evolve we become more intelligent, and as we become more intelligent we give up the less intelligent ways of the past. Knowing what we know today, there is no justification for children under the age of eighteen to engage in high-impact contact sports."

Which for Eric Kluver makes perfect sense theoretically. But emotionally, the solution is not so simple. Take away football from these high school boys, and we as a nation lose something important that's shaped generations of American men.

In the wake of Zac's death, Kluver has changed the way he coaches football. He has drastically decreased the contact in practices. His coaches now teach Hawk tackling, a rugby-style tackle popularized by Seattle Seahawks coach Pete Carroll. It tries to take the head out of the impact of the tackle, as opposed to previous styles of tackling that taught players to get their head out in front. Players are now taught to keep their heads behind, and to avoid slamming their face masks with the ball carrier. In preseason meetings with parents, Kluver stresses the importance of taking concussions seriously, and tells them that any player with a suspected concussion will go through a concussion protocol. "People know Zac's story," Kluver said. "It's the elephant in the room."

The other elephant in the room: Football is violent. It just is. Millions of American boys and young men aren't suddenly going to trade in the cathartic violence of tackle football for the simulacrum that is flag football. The love for the sport would disappear in a flag football world. So instead of the Omalu solution, football tries to improve incrementally, to get safer on the margins while retaining the core element of physical danger and risk that's been central to its appeal since before Theodore Roosevelt.

"No matter how you slice it, it's going to be a contact sport," Kluver said. "I don't know how you change the game while still keeping it similar."

TWO WEEKS AFTER Zac turned the shotgun on himself and pulled the trigger, I met the Easter family for the first time in person, having spoken to Brenda by phone a few days earlier. In the living room—with Zac's ten-point buck mounted to the wall and hovering over us—Zac's father, his mother, his older brother, Ali, Sue Wilson, and I sat in a semicircle. We spoke for almost four hours. There were not many tears, in part because the family was still in shock, and in part because they now had a charge.

In the writings he left behind, Zac gave his family and friends clear instructions: They should not let his death be in vain. His family framed his suicide not as the ultimate selfish act but as something very different: as a sacrifice that meant his death could take on a greater meaning and could be used to help others like him. So the family moved quickly from the stasis of mourning into actually doing something. Starting a foundation in his honor. Speaking to football players about the risk of concussions. Pushing the NFL to take the risks more seriously. Raising money and awareness for research into concussions and CTE. Anything to give a sense of meaning to Zac's senseless death.

How did they feel about football, and the sport's future? Well, it's complicated. Brenda Easter—who had winced back in college when her future husband would get in an on-field collision playing for Drake University and cringed whenever her three sons were involved in crunching hits on the gridiron—was done with the sport. She would put up with it on the television in the living room because this sport was so ingrained in the family's consciousness and history. But there would be zero chance that her grandchildren would play. They could play basketball or baseball or run track instead.

"There was a time when football was instilled in everybody in society," Brenda told me. "In the small towns, that's all they had to do. Football Friday nights is the thing to do. But does that mean that it can't be changed? That something else safer can't replace it?" Her feelings against football, especially for youth, would only harden with time and with more research. Like when she learned about a Harvard study that showed the average white American male lives to age seventy-eight, and the average black American male lives to seventy, but the average professional football player in both the United States and Canada lives to his mid to late fifties. Or when she learned about a study—commissioned by the NFL right around the time Zac was a high school senior and conducted by the University of Michigan's Institute for Social Research—that reported Alzheimer's disease and similar memory-related diseases among NFL retirees were nineteen times the normal rate for men ages thirty to forty-nine. The answer to her felt obvious: Less football would mean safer children.

On a summer night a couple of years after Zac's death, after I had gotten to know the family quite well, I sat at the Easters' kitchen table with Brenda and Myles for hours, drinking beer and talking about Zac and about football. At one point, when I kept pressing Brenda on how she feels about football today, and if the lessons learned from football outweigh the risks of the sport,

Brenda lost her temper with me. "I get angry every day," she told me. "You asked me, 'Do I hate football?' I don't *hate* football. I get angry that the thing that everybody loves is so dangerous. Do I hate the sport? It's a struggle. Because I want to hate the sport so bad. Because it took my son. But I can't. Because I know how much Zac loved it. I know how much all the boys and the fans love it. What I wish is that we could figure out today how to protect them so they can continue to do what they love. The fact I can't protect them, despite knowing what I know today, makes me ill."

For Myles Easter, the guilt was overwhelming. He had pushed his three sons to play the sport, and now his middle one was gone because of it. Yet decades of playing and coaching and watching a specific version of football—the old-school version that exalted the Easter mentality—had formed so much of who Myles Easter was. He still didn't want football to change too much. This was the sport that forged men from boys. It's been a common reaction as long as people have been trying to reform the violence out of football. After a 1931 report by the Carnegie Foundation predicted touch football would replace tackle football, Lone Star Dietz, a former teammate of Jim Thorpe and then the head football coach at Haskell Institute, responded angrily: "They're trying to make a sissy game out of football." Even after all he'd been through, that's still how Myles Easter ultimately felt about his beloved game of football. All these new rules were weakening the sport. He missed the old days. More accurately, he missed the naïve days, when you could play football and coach football and watch football without knowing exactly what those hits to the head were doing to the players' brains.

Ali still recognized how much Zac had adored the sport. But in her mind, football would forever be the thing that killed her boyfriend and changed the trajectory of her life. "I have such a complicated relationship with football," she said. "I feel conflicted. I understand the benefits, and why people love it, but I also know so much needs to change. It's the sport that contributed to my boyfriend's death. What do you do from there?" In the years after his death, Ali would throw herself into fund-raising for scientific research to protect athletes, especially youth athletes, from going down the same road as Zac. She would make frequent visits to the cemetery (the one wish of Zac's they didn't follow). She would bring flowers and a Monster Energy drink, Zac's favorite, and just sit by his memorial headstone and talk with him.

As we spoke in the Easters' living room just weeks after Zac's death, the television was on mute, tuned to the Vikings-Packers. Huge game. Bitter rivals, the NFC North title on the line. As we spoke about Zac's zest for life and Zac's struggles that led to his death, the men in the house, including me, kept peeking at our phones. We were checking our fantasy-football scores.

ZAC LEFT INSTRUCTIONS: Print his story off his laptop, post it to Facebook, use the pain of his life and too-early death to warn the world about CTE. Get people like us—football fans, football players, football parents, football lifers—to face the truth about people like him. And his family did all that, and continues to, through their nonprofit foundation, CTE Hope, dedicated to aiding scientific research to limit and prevent concussions in sports. Ali continues to be a driving force for the foundation, as does Sue Wilson. After graduating magna cum laude from law school and being named a national law student of the year by *National Jurist*, Ali took a job at a corporate law firm in New York City. She's doing the type of high-powered legal work—in her firm's white-collar, investigations, securities litigation, and compliance group—that Zac expected from her. On the side, she coordinates the foundation's communications. She returns to Iowa each year to organize the foundation's spring gala.

Sue Wilson got a taste of public service as vice president of the state's Advisory Council on Brain Injury; in that capacity, she helped develop a brain injury screening tool for places like jails and homeless shelters to determine if mental health issues had been caused by a previous brain injury. Sue then decided to run for a spot on the Indianola School Board on a platform of addressing students' mental health. She won. The woman who a dozen years ago was an unwelcome sight on the Indianola Indians' sidelines has since gained an outsize voice in the community. As one of the cofounders of CTE Hope, Sue spearheaded a research partnership with Myles's alma mater, Drake University. The university is helping develop treatment protocols for people suffering from early symptoms of CTE. The school is also starting a brain injury curriculum in its health sciences department. The classes are geared toward those studying pharmacy, physical therapy, occupational therapy, and athletic training. Sue will be an adjunct professor.

If Zac were around to see the foundation's growth, he'd be thrilled to see how his family, his girlfriend, and his friends followed his instructions. His family and the foundation advocated for legislation for Iowa high schools to update their return-to-play protocol, which was signed by the governor a couple of years after Zac's death. They are also advocating for more controversial nationwide legislation to eliminate tackle football before age fourteen, when a young and developing brain is most susceptible to traumatic brain injury. The foundation launched a saliva research study, which has collected around four thousand saliva samples from football and soccer players statewide and sent them to a research lab at Harvard Medical School. The study aims to measure inflammatory markers and proteins associated with head trauma, with a goal of developing a device, similar to a pregnancy test or a blood-sugar testing device, that can immediately identify a concussion. His family has followed Zac's instructions to a T.

Although he doesn't know the Easter family and hasn't been active in the foundation, Dr. Shawn Spooner has, in his own way, followed Zac's instructions as well. Inspired by Zac and a few other patients who struggled to find timely, quality concussion-related care, he pushed his health-care provider, UnityPoint Health, to build a new facility focused largely on concussion. It's the same model Spooner worked with in Afghanistan, with a large interdisciplinary team—a sports neuropsychologist and a specialty physician, a speech-language pathologist and an athletic trainer and several physical therapists—all under one roof.

But Zac's instructions left no guidance about how to mourn, and no guidance about how we should think about our national sport.

So now what?

We could ban football. (But we love football.) We could allow people to play football only once they turn eighteen, as Omalu has proposed. (OK, but what happens when eighteen-year-old athletic phenoms—freight trains who have never learned to tackle properly—are suddenly turned loose on one another? Would that be *better?*) We could take away tackling. (Sorry, no one's watching the National Flag Football League.) We could build a safer helmet. (Which will only encourage players to use their heads as weapons.) We could have a consistent concussion protocol through all levels of football. (We already do in the NFL.)

Every solution ends up not solving enough of the problem.

And for most of us, this is perfectly OK. The paradox of CTE's discovery is that it's given most of us a sneaky ethical out, hasn't it? No professional football player can claim now to be unaware of the risks. It's a free country. We're all adults here.

Unless we're not adults.

Unless we're kids.

Unless we're Zac.

THE EMAIL ARRIVED in Brenda Easter's Hotmail inbox at 5:33 p.m. on Tuesday, May 24, 2016, five months after Zac had committed suicide. The email was from Bennet Omalu. Shortly after Zac's death, Brenda had shipped Zac's brain to Omalu's old forensic neuropathology lab in Pittsburgh, the same lab that studied Mike Webster's brain. Pathologists had cut Zac's brain into paper-thin slices, put them on slides, and used special chemicals to study whether the buildup of tau proteins in Zac's brain indicated he had CTE.

"Brain Report," Omalu's subject line read. Attached was a PDF document: "Zachary Easter, Brain Forensic Neuropathology Report."

The report was completed by a pathologist named Dr. Julia Kofler and contained plenty of basic details. That Zac had died by suicide in December 2015. That he had played football from age nine until eighteen and sustained multiple confirmed concussions from playing. That his brain weighed 1,540 grams. But right there on the first page of the report, the CTE diagnosis that Zac had feared was confirmed. Tau protein buildup was "widespread" in his brain. The report cited the multiple concussions from football as a potential cause.

Zac was right. The crazy brain disease that had felled famous football players like seventeen-year NFL veteran Mike Webster or twenty-year NFL veteran Junior Seau had, somehow, crept into Zac's brain by the time he was twenty-four. To his parents, the diagnosis brought conflicting emotions. First, it felt impossible. Sure, he was a reckless player, but Zac hadn't even played football past high school.

But, then, the diagnosis also felt strangely comforting. Zac was right all along. If neuropathologists had looked at his brain and seen nothing out of order, his parents would have been doubly devastated. There wouldn't have been an explanation for his death that made any sense. Now, at the very least, they could say they knew what their son was experiencing. The email brought the family a peculiar type of relief.

CAN YOU IMAGINE football just . . . going away?

No more feelings of anticipation as the long days of summer start to wane, and as training camps kick off, and as football openers are right around the corner. No more autumn tableaus of Americana where preteens play raucous, helmetless games of tackle football in yards covered with leaves. No more Thanksgivings spent gathered around the television to watch the Dallas Cowboys or the Detroit Lions. No more Friday night lights, no more Saturday morning tailgates, no more Sundays blanketed with NFL games, no more *NFL Monday Night Football*: A new era in which America simply can no longer stomach the repercussions of this sport.

No more football? No way. Americans have a remarkable capability to compartmentalize our morality. Convincing ourselves that, sure, this sport has obvious negative side effects, and that those negative side effects are far greater than we'd ever imagined but

deciding that we love it anyway. "That's what the NFL is bank-
ing on these next few years—hypocrisy, basically—as more stories
emerge about the tortured lives of retired players," sportswriter Bill
Simmons wrote in the wake of the NFL's Bountygate scandal, with
New Orleans Saints coaches accused of paying out cash bonuses,
or "bounties," for a Saint injuring an opposing player. "You hear
these things, you sigh, you feel remorse, you forget . . . and then
you go back to looking forward to the next football season."

I don't say all this as some self-righteous tut-tutter of America's
football hypocrisy but instead as a full-blown participant in it. I'm
still a hard-core NFL fan. Even as I write this book about how
football played a role in Zac Easter's death—as I interview family members of others who committed suicide after suffering from
football-induced CTE, as I nod in agreement when my wife says
there's zero chance our two young sons, Owen and Lincoln, will
ever play the sport—I still watch.

And it's not some sick addiction that I hide from my family.
I wear it proudly, looking forward to watching NFL games on
Sundays alongside my rambunctious three-year-old son, Lincoln.
Like Zac, our second son is joyous and kind, devious and destructive. "FOOTBAAAAALL!" Lincoln will scream at me, then try to
bowl me over. We've nicknamed him Lincoln the Marauder. It's
only a matter of time before these theoretical discussions between
my wife and me about football become very real, when all Lincoln's
friends are suiting up for the team and he wants to suit up, too.

Omalu diagnoses America's inability to rationally think about
football's future as cognitive dissonance: Our views are shaped by
societal expectations and traditions, and we simply ignore evidence
that goes against those long-held beliefs. "God did not intend for
us to play football," Omalu told me. "Nature, our human bodies,

did not intend for us to expose our heads to repeated blunt force trauma . . . Your child, I guarantee you, has some degree of brain damage if he plays this game for a length of time."

It's a moral problem, yes. But it's a business problem, too; football is a big business. Billionaire owners of NFL teams, major American universities that have staked their public reputations on the sport, small towns that have made shrine-like high school football stadiums among the most important pieces of infrastructure in their town: We're all invested. The sport's tentacles go deep.

"It is possible that football will grow less popular in this country," Steve Almond writes in his book, *Against Football: One Fan's Reluctant Manifesto*. "Here's how it might happen: First, several retired stars might reveal the depth of their neurological impairment. Steve Young on *60 Minutes*. Brett Favre weeping to Oprah. Second, the safer equipment and rules that fans are forever touting as silver bullets may do little to alter the brutal physics of the game. Third, medical technology inevitably will make visible the damage done to young men who play the sport. Fourth, a major college or pro player might be paralyzed or killed during a game. Fifth, a successful class-action suit at the high school or college level could trigger a domino effect."

MYLES EASTER CAN remember, as a kid in the 1960s and 1970s, gathering around the television to watch boxing matches with his father. When Myles's father was growing up, boxing was considered one of our top national sports, "a symbol of American sport," according to a 1944 article in the *Journal of Health and Physical Education*.

But Myles never watched boxing matches with his own sons, perhaps because our society came to deem boxing too primitive, too dangerous, and we lost our collective stomach for it. Boxing still exists, of course, but as a niche sport. There used to be boxing clubs all over American high schools and colleges. Now, those are few and far between. One of the watershed moments of the sport's fall from grace came in 1982, when Howard Cosell, an ABC sportscaster and one of the foremost faces of American boxing for a quarter century, witnessed Larry Holmes beat down Tex Cobb in a bloody, lopsided fight. A couple of weeks before, Ray Mancini had beat down Duk Koo Kim in another bloody, lopsided fight (nationally televised on CBS) that caused Kim to die from brain injuries. Cosell was disgusted; he vowed after the Holmes fight to never call another professional match. "I've had it," Cosell told the *New York Times*. "I now favor the abolition of professional boxing." There have been plenty of ex-football players to offer similar critiques of their sport. Americans have mostly shrugged them off. Ed Cunningham, a former NFL player who was a college football analyst for ESPN and ABC, resigned in 2017 because of his concerns with the sport. Plenty of high-profile NFL players have retired early because of concerns about brain trauma. Perhaps, though, that rejection of football by people who are intimately in its orbit will, in time, reach some sort of tipping point.

"Maybe [football is] popular because it's the one huge cultural space where we can safely indulge all the shit we haven't worked out yet as a people: our lust for violence, our racial neuroses, our yearning for patriarchal dominion, our sexual hang-ups," Almond writes. "It's the place where men get to be boys—before the age of reason, before the age of guilt."

But today, as a society, we're *in* the age of reason, *in* the age of guilt. We can no longer plead ignorance that we simply didn't know what all those hits to the head could do to the human brain. Now, we know. We are no longer innocent bystanders but active participants, complicit in whatever damage football brings. We look back at those old NFL films—*NFL's Greatest Hits* or *Big Blocks and King Size Hits*, *Crunch Course* or *Thunder and Destruction*—as stuff of a prior age. We look back at the old introduction to *Monday Night Football*, with two helmets ramming into each other and exploding, as an unenlightened form of this sport. We cringe when we think about the old ESPN segment, "Jacked Up," in which sportscasters would show a big hit and then chant, "You just got . . . JACKED UP!" We realize that handing out BIG HAMMER T-shirts to high school students to celebrate a punishing hit from a football game probably is not the best practice. We punish the NFL coach for paying his defensive players $1,500 apiece for hits that resulted in opponents being knocked out: "Kill the head, the body will die!" New Orleans Saints defensive coordinator Gregg Williams would tell his players. But then, after being suspended for one season, we welcome that coach back into the league.

We think that we have reformed football. We say that football is safer now than it ever has been. But do we really know how true that is?

There are only two morally upstanding ways to approach the concerns we have about football as our national sport: To devote every resource we have to making it as safe as possible when it comes to brain injuries. Or to renounce the sport completely.

They say that you must hit bottom before you renounce your addiction. What would the bottom look like for a nation addicted to football? Perhaps it could be something spectacular, like a player dying from a massive hit during a nationally televised game. Or it could be something more mundane, like a credible lab test that can use biomarkers to diagnose the onset of CTE in living brain tissue and show an exact percentage of American high school football players who already have incipient CTE.

Think about Myles Easter's all-time favorite player: Jack Tatum, "the Assassin." When a hit by Tatum paralyzed Darryl Stingley in 1978, that could be compartmentalized by the average American football fan. This was a freak hit: unnecessary roughness, not a natural part of the game of football. These types of hits can be legislated out of the sport, and that's exactly what the NFL and every lower form of football has attempted to do in recent years. But what if, like many scientists posit, it may not be those huge, bone-rattling hits that are the primary precursor for CTE but instead the multiple subconcussive hits that occur hundreds of times during every NFL game (and every college game, and every high school game)? Those hits are *necessary* roughness, a routine by-product of how the game is played. An improved concussion protocol won't make a difference for the cases of CTE that stem from years of repeated subconcussive hits. While the notion of football being ostracized by society is today mocked as an idea of the effete, liberal, nanny-state crowd, the social pressures to stop smoking or to wear seat belts were once mocked in much the same way, too. The day may come when parents would be as apt to let their children play football as they are to allow them to ride in a car without a car seat.

But we love violence, right? What if football is recognized as so dangerous that the vast majority of parents won't allow their sons to play, and it becomes our equivalent of gladiatorial combat, only engaged in by the poor and people without options? America's have-nots, going out to the gridiron and destroying themselves for the pleasure of America's haves. Football could become the forbidden fruit, the sport so many are afraid to play—and, perhaps, the game would become even more violent in response. In ancient Rome, gladiators were seen as human sacrifices. Echoes of those gladiators can be heard in the words of former Pittsburgh Steelers running back Rashard Mendenhall, who in 2014 said no thanks to millions more dollars and retired from football at age twenty-six: "I no longer wish to put my body at risk for the sake of entertainment."

So is football worth it? It may be the most important question of our American sporting time. And it's a question without a clean answer. Perhaps it's the story of Zac Easter that can lead us to the most appropriate way to look at football. Zac knew he had CTE. He knew before the doctors did. And he blamed football, and the concussions he suffered while playing the sport. At times, he hated everything about the sport. At times, though, he loved the sport as much as just about anything in his life. Even after knowing what the sport and the way he approached the sport had done to his brain, even after the very public suicide attempt that landed him in the psych ward, there Zac was, sitting in his parents' basement on Thanksgiving night, watching his beloved Green Bay Packers.

Football is awful, a sport that brings out the very worst violent tendencies in the human species, and that destroys us in the process.

Football is great, the one true sport, teaching us how to deal with physical pain without being utterly defeated by it while forging the true American male.

Football is a dangerous, vile sport. Football is a beautiful, cathartic sport.

Football, perhaps, is both.

A WEEK AFTER Zac's death, on Ali's twenty-third birthday, Brenda Easter handed her an envelope. Inside was $1,400, the money from Zac's final paycheck for a landscaping job. He had left instructions that it go to Ali. Zac hadn't been working for a while, so this underscored to Ali just how purposeful his suicide had been—that he'd been planning it for a long time.

In the months after his death, Ali began to think of herself as a widow; even though they hadn't been married, they'd been best friends for five years, and dated off and on that entire period, so labeling herself as a widow felt morbidly appropriate. Ali went to a jewelry store and designed a ring. It had five stones. Two were pearls—Zac's birthstone—and three were blue sapphires, their shared favorite color. On the inside of the ring was inscribed, *Z+W*, for *Zac+Winslow*. She thought of it as their wedding ring of sorts. They'd been planning to spend their lives together. The ring represented what could have been.

For Christmas 2016, one year after Zac's death, Ali made some presents for Zac's parents and brothers—picture frames engraved with Zac's handwriting and personalized football sweatshirts for each of them: Vikings sweatshirts for Myles Sr. and Myles II, a Chiefs sweatshirt for Levi, a Packers sweatshirt for Brenda. The back of each sweatshirt read EASTER, with Zac's old football number, 44.

After buying the ring, Ali still had some of Zac's money left over. So on December 23, 2016, when she was home for winter break of her second year in law school, Ali and Jake Powers, Zac's old friend and roommate, got in Jake's truck at the crack of dawn and drove east. They passed through the cornfields of Iowa, crossed the Mississippi River at Dubuque, headed northeast through Wisconsin, and came to a halt seven hours later in Green Bay, Wisconsin, for the Packers' final home game of the 2016 regular season. For Ali, it was a trip full of complicated emotions. Lambeau Field was one of Zac's favorite places on Earth,

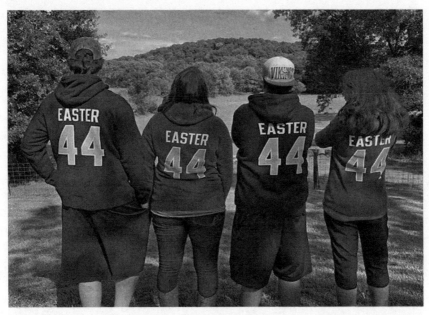

The Easter family timber; the ridge where Zac shot his 10-point buck is in the distance. From left: Levi, Ali, Myles II, Brenda.

a cathedral of football. He'd been there only once, in December 2014, for the first Packers game he'd ever attended. Zac came back from that trip inspired to turn that into an annual tradition with Jake. Ali wanted to be there in Zac's place, even if that meant paying homage to the sport that had contributed to his destruction.

The next day, Christmas Eve, they went to Lambeau Field, first to the massive tailgate and then to the game. Ali wore her Packers sweatshirt with Zac's name and number on the back. She wore Zac's old Packers knit cap.

Ali's feelings about football are nuanced. She recognizes it is something that brings people together, and that has many positive influences in people's lives. But she is angry that football—that the NFL—took so long to recognize the damage the sport can cause.

The disregard felt like a betrayal of the very people it employs and entertains. Still, Ali wanted to see Lambeau, and she wanted to cheer on the Packers in place of Zac, even if that meant honoring the thing she believes killed him. If Zac had lived, he would have been here with her, reliving his memories of his beloved Packers. So she yelled wildly as the Packers beat the Vikings, 38–25, and eliminated their archrivals from the playoff race. It was easy to get lost in the excitement, in the tradition, in the history, even if every time a player endured a hard hit to the head, Ali winced.

This, Ali felt, was the way Zac would have wanted to be honored. Yes, Zac had grown to hate what football had done to him. But the sport had been such a big part of his life: being a man whose character was formed through football, having heroes, believing in something. Ali thought these football pilgrimages could be a way to keep Zac's spirit alive, and to keep their love alive, too.

After the game, she and Jake got in his truck and drove back to Iowa. Ali fell asleep. They got home just before midnight on Christmas Eve. During the drive, Ali felt Zac was right there alongside them.

Epilogue

The final words of Zac Easter's autobiography:

To my family,

I just want everyone in my family to know that I love them dearly and to not dwell on my death. I have been thinking about this for years now and there is truly nothing anyone could have done to prevent this. I have spent many nights speaking to God and I know that my spirit will live on in rejoice. The lord understands my pain and has accepted me to be one of his children. I ask that no one blame themselves for anything that I have been through. There is nothing you could of done to help me. It has been my choice. I know how it works and I know that a lot of family members will feel a terrible burden and feel that they should have known or should have tried to help. I ask that you all come together and try to spread the word of the dangers of head injuries and mental health. I ask that we can all get along and become closer as a family. You may cry, but just know that I will be always watching over you and will be with you at every holiday, and any moment that you need me in your life. Just look to the lord and pray, and I will be there

to guide you through anything difficult that you may be facing. This goes for all friends and family. I ask that you do
not feel guilty or blame each other! Do not blame football
or specifically anything that had to do with me. Just know
that I enjoyed playing through it and after fighting through
it all, I still consider myself to be one of the toughest people
I know. IT IS NOT YOUR FAULT. I love all of you and hold
no grudges. If only you all knew how guilty and ashamed I
feel for taking the easy way out.

Mom and Dad, I love you both dearly and I am truly
sorry that one of your sons has passed before his time. I
loved both of you dearly and there is nothing you could of
done parenting wise to prevent this. I know that both of you
will mourn naturally over the loss of your son, but just know
that I am in a place where I am free of the pain. I have spent
many nights talking to the lord and I my spirit will be fine.
The lord understands my situation and has accepted me into
his open arms. I have spent many nights talking to the lord
about how truly I am blessed to have parents like you both.
Through the good and bad, you two have been there for me
through thick and thin. You both worked your asses off to
provide for me and I am forever thankful to have parents to
teach me such strong values growing up. I have had it much
better than anyone I know. You have taught me so much
about life and I don't regret any of the moments we've spent
together. You both taught me right from wrong and how
nothing is earned without a strong work ethic. I hope that
you guys don't ever feel guilty for what I have done. It is not
your fault, if it was, you know I'm the type of asshole who
would tell you . . . Whatever has happened to me is not your

fault. It is what is. Do not dwell for the lord has better plans for all of us.

To my brothers, I love you two both more than anything and I know this will be tough for you two to handle the most. We have always been brothers through thick and thin. We've fought some pretty intense fights in the past and have strengthened the bond over the years. I couldn't never have been more proud to say that both Levi and Myles are my brothers. The Easter boys have certainly raised hell through the years and I wouldn't change a minute of it! We've lived some of the sickest times together and have been through things I wouldn't change for a minute. I know both of you are destined to do great things in your own realms. I know both of you will change the world in your own ways. Your both destined for greatness. You may not see it in this time of mourning, but I promise God has a strong purpose for both of you. Please do not morn my death, instead embrace it. Just know that Zac will always be overhead watching over you guys as you carry out your dreams. Don't be scared to ask for help when times get rough because they will. Just know that I will always be over guys shoulder looking out for you and God's always got your back. When you call, I will be there, I will help you make it through the long days and dark nights. Have faith, be your own men, keep fighting, and never quit. I look up to both of you for being warriors and fighting through any adversity that may come upon you. I truly am sorry for any times I have said things to make you feel down or feel bad. Just remember me the person I am, not by my actions. I'm not sure what is wrong with me and people will figure it out eventually. Just know that I love you both and I will always be therefore you. Live your lives with no regrets. Get tattoos. Spend your money on drugs and hoes. I will be living those moments with you guys and will never leave you alone. Spread the word of mental illness and concussions. Do great things and know I always have your back. Keep fighting through and good things will happen, and Never ever forget, Zac will have your back. The shame still haunts me of certain times when I was dicks to you guys and made you feel like I was superior, please forgive me for the times I was an asshole. We've all seen different sides of Zac and I hope you remember the times when I was actually Zac and not the asshole one who made anyone feel shitty about themselves.

Forever family

I am terribly sorry for my decision. I have taken the easy way out and have taken the most shameful coarse of action. It brings tears to my eyes thinking about the good times we've had. I can't stop thinking about something has changed in me and I don't know what it is. I ask to have my brain donated to the Sports Legacy Brain Bank.

I don't know what has changed in me, whether it be mental illness or something more from the concussions. All I ask is that you please donate my brain to the sports legacy brain bank to try and find out. What ever it be take it with grace and know I love you all. Spread the word of mental illness and concussions, and over time, please spread my story. Great things can still happen from this event. Think of all the lives that can be saved if all of you come together and help people by spreading the word.

Acknowledgments

THIS BOOK WOULD not have been possible without the indomitable courage of Zac Easter's family and those closest to him, specifically his parents, Brenda and Myles Sr.; his brothers, Myles II and Levi; and his girlfriend, Alison Epperson. For them to allow me to document the pain they all experienced in the immediate aftermath of Zac's death—and for them to share with me Zac's most personal thoughts and writings—took an enormous amount of bravery, as well as trust. I can hope only that this book faithfully portrays the young man they knew and loved.

So many friends, relatives, and acquaintances of Zac spoke with me as I researched, wrote, and revised this book: Sue Wilson, Eric Kluver, Shawn Spooner, Kamela Kleppe-Yeager, Jake Powers, Nick Haworth, Father Jacob Greiner, Mike Hadden, Ryan Miller, Chase Wells, and many others. Their memories helped paint a full portrait of Zac.

The scientific experts, the historians, and the activists: From their writings and research, as well as from my own one-on-one interviews, I've learned so much about football, about the history of the concept of masculinity, about brain science, and about the efforts to mitigate the effects of head trauma. In no particular order, I owe much gratitude to: Bennet Omalu, Cyndy Feasel, Dominic

Malcolm, Tom Oates, Michael Oriard, Jeanne Marie Laskas, Gerald R. Gems, Michael MacCambridge, Michael Sokolove, Kimberly Archie, Debra Pyka, Kevin Bieniek, Randy Benson, Ann McKee, Gary Swenson, Frank Salamone, Dawn Goodale, Joey Goodale, Mary Seau, Alan Sills, Kevin Guskiewicz, Mike McCrea, Jason Mihalik, Adam Bartsch, and others.

Every story needs a great editor. This book was blessed with several: Devin Gordon, who saw something powerful in my blind submission and (brilliantly, patiently) shepherded the original story from just an idea to its publication in *GQ* in January 2017. Markus Hoffmann, my literary agent, who showed me, a would-be book author, how to write a successful book proposal. It was Debbie Spander, my media agent, who connected me with Markus. My collaborators at Algonquin were perfect: Amy Gash believed in the book from the beginning and trusted me to write it. Margot Herrera's gifts as an editor made this book infinitely better. Robin Cruise's careful attention to wordcraft and typos was crucial. In addition, my wife, Megan—who is always my first and my last editor—was steadfast every step of the way.

The patience and support of my wife and children was invaluable during this years-long process. My parents nurtured a love of reading in me dating from my birth. My best friend, Bill Reiter, became my writing mentor. I'm indebted to him and many more mentors along the way, including the late, great Ken Fuson.

Lastly, this book never would have come to be without the foresight and, yes, courage of Zac Easter. The nasty stew of mental illness and concussion-related issues that led to Zac's demise represents a vital concern in today's America. My intent for telling Zac's story is not to glorify his suicide; his own words underscore the shame and regret Zac's decision caused him. But I believe that once Zac made the decision his life was too painful for him to continue, he had come to think of himself as a sacrifice—and he hoped that his story could help others who lived after him. I too can only hope that it will.